AF835763

*A Garland Series*

# British Philosophers and Theologians of the 17th & 18th Centuries

A Collection of 101 Volumes

Edited by

René Wellek

# Joseph Priestley

## AN EXAMINATION
## 1774

Garland Publishing, Inc., New York & London

1978

Bibliographical note:

this facsimile has been made from a copy in the
Yale University Library
(K8.P93b774)

**Library of Congress Cataloging in Publication Data**

Priestley, Joseph, 1733-1804.
An examination, 1774.

(British philosophers and theologians of the 17th & 18th centuries)
Reprint of the 1774 ed. printed for J. Johnson, London, under title: An examination of Dr. Reid's Inquiry into the human mind on the principles of common sense, Dr. Beattie's Essay on the nature and immutability of truth, and Dr. Oswald's Appeal to common sense in behalf of religion.
1. Philosophy, Scottish. 2. Reid, Thomas, 1710-1796. Inquiry into the human mind. 3. Beattie, James, 1735-1803. Essay on the nature and immutability of truth. 4. Oswald, James, d. 1793. An appeal to common sense. 5. Senses and sensation. 6. Truth. 7. Apologetics--18th century. 8. Skepticism--Controversial literature. I. Title. II. Series.
B1401.P9 1978 111.8'3 75-11249
ISBN 0-8240-1800-1

*Printed in the United States of America*

# AN
# EXAMINATION
## OF

Dr. REID'S *Inquiry into the Human Mind on the Principles of Common Senſe,*

Dr. BEATTIE'S *Eſſay on the Nature and Immutability of Truth,*

AND

Dr. OSWALD'S *Appeal to Common Senſe in Behalf of Religion.*

---

By JOSEPH PRIESTLEY, LL. D. F. R. S.

---

*As ſome men have imagined* innate ideas, *becauſe they had forgot how they came by them; ſo others have ſet up almoſt as many* diſtinct inſtincts *as there are* acquired principles *of acting.*

Preliminary Diſſertation to Law's tranſlation of King's Origin of Evil.

---

LONDON:

PRINTED FOR J. JOHNSON, Nº. 72, ST. PAUL'S CHURCH-YARD.

M.DCC.LXXIV.

*To Dr.* REID, *Dr.* BEATTIE, *and* *Dr.* OSWALD.

GENTLEMEN,

I Take the liberty to preſent each of you with a copy of my remarks on your writings, requeſting that you would give them that attention which, according to your own ideas, the ſubject deſerves.

You cannot be juſtly offended at me for treating you with the ſame freedom with which you have treated others. If the public voice, which has hitherto ſeemed to incline to your ſide, ſhould, notwithſtanding, finally determine in my favour, you will be conſidered as bold and insolent innovators in what has hitherto been the received doctrine concerning *human nature*, and in the fundamental principles of *truth* and *reason*. But if your tenets be admitted, and my objections to them be deemed frivolous, I must be content to cover my head with infamy, and fall under the indelible disgrace of a weak or wicked opposer of new and important truth.

I should not have written this book, Gentlemen, if I had not meant to call you forth to defend the ground which you have boldly seized and occupied. It is, therefore, my expectation, and my wish, that you would all of you, either jointly or separately, enter into an open and free discussion

of

of the queſtions which are now before the public. I promiſe to proceed with equal *fairneſs* and *freedom*, acknowledging, with the greateſt frankneſs, any miſtakes or overſights of which I ſhall be convinced; and, judging by your profeſſed liberality and candour, I and the public ſhall expect the ſame conduct from you.

Sincerely wiſhing you all poſſible ſucceſs in your laudable endeavours to ſerve the cauſe of *truth*, *virtue*, and *religion*, though my writings, and myſelf, ſhould be the victims at their ſhrine,

I am, GENTLEMEN,

Your moſt obedient

humble ſervant,

J. PRIESTLEY.

*Calne, Auguſt* 10, 1774.

THE

THE

# PREFACE.

NOTHING could be more unexpected by me, but a very few months ago, than this publication. *Dr. Reid's Inquiry into the principles of the human mind* fell into my hands presently after the first publication of it; but being at that time intent upon my electrical pursuits, and others of a similar nature, I did no more than look very slightly into it. Finding his notions of human nature the very reverse of those which I had learned from Mr. Locke and Dr. Hartley (in which I thought I had sufficient reason to acquiesce) I did not give myself the trouble to read the book through.

It appeared to me to be an ingenious piece of sophistry, and had it been written for the purpoſe of *amuſement*, I might have been pleaſed with it; but I own I was rather ſurprized to ſee ſuch a production uſhered into the world with great gravity, by a profeſſor in a public univerſity; and I was more ſurprized to find that the work was very ſeriouſly admired both in Scotland and England. Afterwards a friend of mine referred me to Dr. Reid's treatiſe for ſome obſervations on the ſubject of *ſquinting*, which I read, and quoted in my *Hiſtory of Optics*; but I did not at that time look any farther into the book than the paſſages to which my friend had directed me.

*Dr. Beattie*'s *Eſſay on Truth* I read through at its firſt coming out, and though his principles appeared to me to be very wrong, I was much pleaſed with the good intention with which the book ſeemed to have been written, and with ſome of his lively ſtrictures upon Mr. Hume; but I had not the moſt diſtant thought of animadverting upon it.

*Dr.*

*Dr. Oswald's Appeal to common sense,* I believe, I should never have heard of, if I had not been referred to it by the author of the *Remarks on my publications.* This, therefore, I procured, but I hardly so much as looked into it, till after the publication of the second volume of my *Institutes of Natural and Revealed Religion;* when, finding the work quoted with much respect by Dr. Beattie and others, and hearing it in general well spoken of, I was determined to give it a careful reading; which I did with great astonishment and indignation, but not without some entertainment.

Unaccountable as it appeared to me that such a performance should ever have excited any other sentiments than those of contempt, in any person who had been initiated into the elements of this kind of knowledge by Mr. Locke, and who entertained any opinion of the *defenceableness of his religion,* I thought it might not be amiss to make a few remarks upon it, in a short *Essay,* which I might prefix to the third volume of my *Inſtitutes.* And there would have been a ſufficient propriety in it; becauſe, if this new ſcheme of an immediate appeal to *common ſenſe* upon every important queſtion in religion (and which ſuperſeded almoſt all *reaſoning* on the ſubject) ſhould take place, the plan of my work, with which I had taken ſome pains, and which I hoped would be of ſome uſe to young perſons, was abſurd from the very beginning.

Accordingly I made ſome notes upon Dr. Oſwald's treatiſe with this view; but finding that I had entered upon a copious, amuſing, and not uninſtructive ſubject, I determined to conſider it more at large. I therefore contented myſelf with a few general remarks upon the ſubject, and an extract or two from Dr. Oſwald, in the preface to that third volume, juſt to give ſome idea of the nature and ſpirit of the principles I meant to oppoſe; promiſing to diſcuſs the ſubject more at large in a ſeparate work, in which I might

alſo

alſo take ſome notice of Dr. Reid, who firſt advanced the principles of which Dr. Beattie and Dr. Oſwald had made ſo much uſe. This has produced the preſent publication, in which I have introduced ſeveral of the remarks and quotations contained in the above-mentioned *preface*; ſuppoſing that, as this work is of a very different nature from that, the ſame perſons might not be poſſeſſed of them both.

Thinking farther upon this ſubject, it occurred to me, that the moſt effectual method to divert the attention of the more ſenſible part of the public from ſuch an incoherent ſcheme as that of Dr. Reid, and to eſtabliſh the true ſcience of human nature, would be to facilitate the ſtudy of *Dr. Hartley*'s *Theory*. I therefore communicated my deſign to the ſon of that extraordinary man, who was pleaſed to approve of my undertaking. Accordingly I have now in the preſs an edition of ſo much of the *Obſervations on Man* as relate to the doctrine of aſſoci-

ation

ation of ideas, leaving out the doctrine of *vibrations*, and some other things which might discourage many readers; and introducing it with some dissertations of my own.

Also, to show the great importance and extensive use of this excellent theory of the mind, I thought it might be of service to give some specimens of the application of Dr. Hartley's doctrine to such subjects of inquiry as it had a near relation to, and to which I had had occasion to give particular attention. And as I had, on other accounts, been frequently requested to publish the *Lectures on Philosophical Criticism*, which I composed when I was tutor in the Belles Lettres at the academy at Warrington, this was another inducement to the publication. For it appears to me that the subject of criticism admits of the happiest illustration from Dr. Hartley's principles; and accordingly, in the composition of those lectures, I kept them continually in view.

But

But the moſt important application of Dr. Hartley's doctrine of the aſſociation of ideas is to *the conduct of human life*, and eſpecially the buſineſs of *education*. I therefore propoſe to publiſh ſome obſervations on this ſubject, perhaps pretty ſoon; and I ſhall reſerve for a time of more leiſure, and more advanced age, the throwing together and ſyſtematizing the obſervations that I am from time to time making on the general conduct of *human life* and *happineſs*, and on the natural *progreſs and perfection of intellectual beings*.

This work, if I be able, in any tolerable meaſure, to accompliſh my deſign, will contain not merely *illuſtrations*, and the moſt important *applications* of Hartley's theory, but may contribute in ſome meaſure to the *improvement* and *extenſion* of it. Speculations of this kind contribute to my own entertainment and happineſs almoſt every day of my life; and were philoſophers in general to attend to them, they would find in them an inexhauſtible

hauſtible fund of diſquiſition, abounding with the moſt excellent practical uſes; more eſpecially inſpiring the greateſt elevation of thought, continually leading the mind to views beyond the narrow limits of the preſent ſtate, and filling it with the pureſt ſentiments of benevolence and devotion.

I am fully aware how exceedingly unpopular ſome of the opinions advanced in this work will be, not with the vulgar only, but alſo with many ingenious and excellent perſons, for whom I have the higheſt eſteem, and who are diſpoſed to think favourably of my other publications. But as they have not diſapproved of my uſual freedom in avowing and defending opinions in which they concur with me; I hope they will bear with the ſame *uniform freedom*, and love of truth, though it ſhould lead me to adopt and aſſert opinions in which they cannot give me their concurrence.

As

As to the doctrine of *neceſſity*, to which I now principally refer, it may poſſibly ſave ſome perſons, who will think that I would not ſpeak at random, not a little trouble, if I here give it as my opinion, that unleſs they apply themſelves to the ſtudy of this queſtion pretty early in life, and in a regular ſtudy of Pneumatology and Ethics, they will never truly underſtand the ſubject; but will always be liable to be impoſed upon, ſtaggered, confounded, and terrified, by the repreſentations of the generality of writers, who, how ſpeciouſly ſoever they declaim, in reality know no more about it than themſelves. The common Arminian doctrine of *free will*, in the only ſenſe of the words in which mankind generally uſe them, viz. *the power of doing what we pleaſe*, or *will*, is the doctrine of the ſcriptures, and is what the philoſophical doctrine of neceſſity ſuppoſes; and farther than this no man does, or need to look, in the common conduct of life, or of religion.

If

If any perſon, at a proper time of life, with his mind diveſted of vulgar prejudices, poſſeſſed of the neceſſary preparatory knowledge, and likewiſe of ſome degree of *fortitude*, which is certainly requiſite for the ſteady contemplation of great and intereſting ſubjects, ſhould chuſe to inquire ſeriouſly into this buſineſs, I would recommend to him, beſides the *ſtudy* (for the *peruſal* is ſaying and doing nothing at all) of Dr. Hartley's Obſervations on man, Mr. *Jonathan Edwards's treatiſe on free will.* This writer diſcuſſes the ſubject with great clearneſs and judgment, obviating every ſhadow of objection to it; and, in my opinion, his work is unanſwerable. But the concurrence of the philoſophical doctrine of *neceſſity* with the gloomy notions of Calvin appears to me to be a ſtrange kind of phenomenon; and I cannot help thinking that had this ingenious writer lived a little longer, and reflected upon the natural connection and tendency of his ſentiments, as explained in his treatiſe, he could not

but

but have ſeen things in a very different light, and have been ſenſible that his philoſophy was much more nearly allied to Socinianiſm than to Calviniſm.

In reality, I can hardly help thinking it to have been a piece of artifice in Mr. Edwards to repreſent the doctrine of philoſophical neceſſity as being the ſame thing with Calviniſm, and the doctrine of philoſophical liberty as the ſame thing with Arminianiſm. Both Arminians and Calviniſts had certainly the very ſame opinion concerning the freedom of the human will in general, though they differed in their notions of it where religion was concerned. In fact, the modern queſtion of *liberty and neceſſity* is what thoſe divines never underſtood, or indeed had ſo much as heard of. The Arminians maintained, in general, that it depends upon men themſelves whether they will be ſaved or not, and the Calviniſts maintained the contrary opinion, aſſerting that it depends wholly upon an arbitrary decree of God. At leaſt, this was the caſe till, in the courſe of the controverſy, they were led to refine upon the ſubject, and at length Mr. Edwards hit upon the true philoſophical doctrine of *neceſſity*, which I ſcruple not to aſſert, that no other Calviniſt ever did before.

Zealous Calviniſts, who regard my writings with abhorrence, will be ſurprized to hear me ſo full and earneſt in my recommendation of a book which they themſelves boaſt of, as the ſtrongeſt bulwark of their own gloomy faith. And they muſt continue to wonder, as it would be to no purpoſe for me to explain to them why they ought not to wonder at the matter. What I ſhould ſay on that ſubject would not be intelligible to them.

Thoſe who are not fond of much cloſe thinking, which is neceſſarily the caſe with the generality of readers, and ſome writers, will not thank me for endeavouring to introduce into more public notice ſuch a theory of the human mind as that of Dr. Hartley. His is not a book that a man can read over in a few evenings, ſo as to be ready to give a ſatiſfactory account of it to any of his friends who may happen to aſk him what there is in it, and expect an anſwer in a few ſentences. In fact, it contains a new and moſt extenſive *ſcience*, and requires a vaſt fund of preparatory knowledge to enter upon the ſtudy of it with any proſpect of ſucceſs.

But, in return, I will promiſe any perſon who ſhall apply to this work, with proper furniture, that the ſtudy of it will abundantly reward his labour. It will be like entering upon *a new world*, afford inexhauſtible matter for curious and uſeful ſpeculation, and be of unſpeakable advantage in almoſt every purſuit, and even in things to which it ſeems, at firſt ſight, to bear no ſort of relation. For my own part, I can almoſt ſay, that I think myſelf more indebted to this one treatiſe, than to all the books I ever read beſide; the ſcriptures excepted.

On the other hand, ſuch a theory of the human mind as that of Dr. Reid, adopted by Dr. Beattie and Dr. Oſwald (if that can be called a *theory* which in fact *explains* nothing) does not, indeed, require much ſtudy; but when you have given all poſſible attention to it, you find yourſelf no wiſer than before. Dr. Reid meets with a particular ſentiment, or perſuaſion, and not being able to explain the origin of it, without more ado he aſcribes it to *a particular original inſtinct,* provided for that very purpoſe. He finds another difficulty, which he alſo ſolves in the ſame conciſe and eaſy manner. And thus he goes on accounting for every thing, by telling you, not only that he cannot explain it himſelf, but that it will be in vain for you, or any other perſon, to endeavour to inveſtigate it farther than he has done. Thus avowed ignorance is to paſs for real knowledge, and, as with the old Sceptics, that man is to be reckoned the greateſt philoſopher who aſſerts that he knows nothing himſelf, and can perſuade others that they know no more than

than he does. There is this difference between the antient and theſe modern ſceptics, that the antients profeſſed neither to *underſtand* nor *believe* any thing, whereas theſe moderns believe every thing, though they profeſs to underſtand nothing. And the former, I think, are the more conſiſtent of the two.

Thoſe of my readers who have not been much converſant with metaphyſical writers, and are not acquainted with the artful manner in which ſome of them draw conſequences from their doctrines, in order to inhance the value of their ſpeculations, cannot poſſibly be aware how much, in the opinion of thoſe whoſe ſentiments I am oppoſing, depends upon the controverſy in which I am now engaged. I ſhall, therefore, in order to excite his attention to the ſubject (beſides what I have obſerved of this nature in the body of the work) quote a few paſſages from Dr. Reid's *Dedication*, which ſhow what important ſervice he imagined he was doing to mankind by his performance; and his diſciples Dr. Beattie and

Dr. Oswald are not behind their master, in the ideas they entertain of the value of their respective writings.

He begins with observing, p. 3, that, though the subject of it had been canvassed by men of very great penetration and genius such as Descartes, Malebranche, Locke, Berkley, and Hume; yet he has given a view of the human understanding so very different from them, as to be apprehensive of being condemned by many for his temerity and vanity. p. 4.

A whole system of scepticism, he says, p. 5, has been fairly built upon the principles of Mr. Locke. Then he observes, p. 6, that if all belief be laid aside, piety, patriotism, friendship, parental affection, and private virtue appear as ridiculous as knight errantry. Upon the hypothesis that he combats, he says, p. 8, the whole universe about him, body and spirit, sun, moon, stars, and earth, friends and relations, all things without exception, vanish at once, and, *like the baseless*

*fabrick*

*fabrick of a vision, leave not a track behind.* He therefore informs his patron, that he thought it unreasonable, upon the authority of philosophers, to admit an hypothesis, which, in his opinion, overturned all philosophy, all religion, and virtue, and common sense. And finding that all the systems concerning the human understanding that he was acquainted with were built upon this hypothesis, he was resolved to inquire into the subject anew, without regard to any hypothesis; and the leisure of an academical life, p. 10, disengaged from the pursuits of interest and ambition, the duty of his profession, which obliged him to give prelections on these subjects to youth, and an early inclination to speculations of this kind, enabled him, he flatters himself, to give a more minute attention to the subject of this inquiry, than had been given before.

He concludes with hinting to his patron, p. 11, who, with many others, had approved of his sentiments, that in it he has juſtified the common ſenſe and reaſon of mankind, againſt the ſceptical ſubtilties which, in this age, have endeavoured to put them out of countenance, and to throw new light upon one of the nobleſt parts of the divine workmanſhip; and therefore that his Lordſhip's reſpect for the arts and ſciences, and his attention to the improvement of them, as well as to every thing elſe that contributes to the felicity of his country, leaves him no room to doubt of his favourable acceptance of his Eſſay.

According to this view of the ſubject, the intereſt and happineſs of mankind are nearly concerned in this buſineſs; and therefore it behoves me to proceed with the greateſt caution. If I deprive the world of the benefit of Dr. Reid's important ſervices, I do them an irreparable injury; but, on the other hand, if I undeceive them with reſpect to the confidence they have been induced to put in one, who, notwithſtanding his profeſſions, in which I doubt not he is very ſincere,

cannot

cannot in reality be of any uſe to them, I ſhall be intitled to ſome portion of their gratitude, though I ſhould confer upon them no poſitive benefit.

I have a ſlight apology to make to thoſe perſons who have not read the writings on which I have animadverted, for the *freedom* with which I have ſometimes treated them. Thoſe who have read them, and have obſerved the airs of ſelf-ſufficiency, arrogance, and contempt of all others who have treated, or touched upon, theſe ſubjects before them, and the frightful conſequences which they perpetually aſcribe to the opinions they controvert (and which are generally my own favourite opinions) will think me to have been very temperate in the uſe that I have made of ſuch a mode of writing, as tends to render metaphyſical ſpeculation not quite tedious, inſipid, and diſguſting. At moſt I have treated them as they have treated others, far ſuperior to themſelves.

As

As to Dr. Ofwald, whom I have treated with the leaft ceremony, the difguft his writings gave me was fo great, that I could not poffibly fhew him more refpect. Indeed I think him in general not intitled to a grave anfwer; and accordingly have for the moft part contented myfelf with *exhibiting* his fentiments, without *replying* to them at all. This will probably confirm him in the opinion which he has already expreffed, viz. that *he fees I have not ftudied the fubject of this controverfy.*

As my remarks on thefe three writers are neceffarily mifcellaneous, I thought it would not be improper to prefix to them a *preliminary effay*, on the nature of judgment and reafoning, with a general view of the progrefs of the intellect, efpecially with refpect to our knowledge of the external world. By this means I hope my reader will enter upon the *particular remarks* with the advantage of a pretty good general knowledge of the fubject; but for a more particular knowledge of it, I muft refer him to the edition of Hartley

above-

above-mentioned, and the diſſertations that I propoſe to prefix to it.

Some may wonder that I ſhould be ſo ſevere on theſe three chriſtian writers, and take no notice of Mr. Hume, whoſe ſophiſtry, being deemed by them to be unanſwerable on the common principles, compelled them to have recourſe to theſe new ones. And others may even think it wrong that, being a chriſtian myſelf, I ſhould not join the triumph of my friends, though the victory was not gained with my weapons.

To the former I anſwer, that, in my opinion, Mr. Hume has been very ably anſwered, again and again, upon more ſolid principles than thoſe of this new common ſenſe; and I beg leave to refer them to the two firſt volumes of my *Inſtitutes* above mentioned, and eſpecially the ſecond, which relates to the evidences of chriſtianity. Beſides, though I have not, in this treatiſe, anſwered Mr. Hume directly, I have done it, in ſome meaſure,

*indirectly,*

*indirectly*, when I ſhow that there was no occaſion to have recourſe to this new mode of defending religion, the old being abundantly ſufficient.

To the latter I would reply, that I reſpect chriſtianity chiefly as it is the cauſe of *truth*, and that the true intereſt of chriſtianity is promoted no leſs by throwing down weak and rotten ſupports, than by ſupplying it with firm and good ones.

After I had announced my intention to animadvert upon Dr. Reid, Dr. Beattie, and Dr. Oſwald, I was told of an anonymous pamphlet, written to ſhow that Dr. Beattie's Eſſay on Truth is *ſophiſtical, and promotive of ſcepticiſm and infidelity*. Though I do not approve of what ſeems to have been the deſign of this writer, I think his remarks are, in the main, juſt with reſpect to Dr. Beattie. My obſervations are frequently the ſame with his.

It is neceſſary for the ſake of verifying my quotations to obſerve that I have made

made uſe of *Dr. Reid's Inquiry*, third edition, London, 1769; *Dr. Beattie's Eſſay*, fifth edition, London, 1774; and *Dr. Oſwald's Appeal*, vol. 1, ſecond edition, London, 1768; vol. 2, the firſt edition, Edinburgh, 1772; *Dr. Price's Review*, ſecond edition, London, 1769; *Harris's Hermes*, London, 1751.

When no particular volume of Dr. Oſwald is expreſſed, the firſt is always intended.

THE

THE

# CONTENTS.

## *Remarks on Dr.* Reid's *Theory.*



SEC-

## SECTION IV.



## SECTION V.



## SECTION VI.



## SECTION VII.



## SECTION VIII.



SEC-

## SECTION IX.



## SECTION X.



## SECTION XI.



## SECTION XII.



## SECTION XIII.



## *Remarks on Dr.* Beattie's *Eſſay.*



SEC-

SECTION I.



SECTION II.



SECTION III.



SECTION IV.



SECTION V.



SECTION VI.



SEC-

*Introductory Obſervations on the nature of* judgment *and* reaſoning, *with a general view of the* progreſs of the Intellect, *with reſpect to the principal ſubjects of this treatiſe.*

WHEN our minds are firſt expoſed to the influence of external objects, all their parts and properties, and even accidental variable adjuncts, are preſented to our view at the ſame time; ſo that the whole makes but one impreſſion upon our organs of ſenſe, and conſequently upon the mind. By this means all the parts of the ſimultaneous impreſſion are ſo intimately aſſociated together, that the idea of any one of them introduces the idea of all the reſt. But as the neceſſary parts and properties will occur more often than the variable adjuncts, the ideas of theſe will not be ſo perfectly aſſociated with the reſt; and thus we ſhall be able to diſtinguiſh between thoſe parts or pro-

 perties

perties that have been found ſeparate, and thoſe that have never been obſerved aſunder.

The idea of any thing, and of its neceſſary inſeparable properties, as thoſe of *milk* and *whiteneſs*, *gold* and *yellow*, always occurring together, is the foundation of, and ſupplies the materials for *propoſitions*, in which they are affirmed of one another, and are *ſaid* to be inſeparable; or, to uſe the terms of logic, in which one is made the *ſubject*, and the other the *predicate* of a propoſition; and nothing is requiſite but *words* to denote the names of things and properties, and any arbitrary ſign for a *copula*, and the propoſition is complete; as *milk is white, gold is yellow, or milk has whiteneſs, gold has yellowneſs*. This claſs of truths contains thoſe in which there is an univerſal, and therefore a ſuppoſed neceſſary connection between the ſubject and the predicate.

Another claſs of truths contains thoſe in which the ſubject and predicate appear,

upon

upon comparifon, to be, in reality, nothing more than different names for the fame thing. To this clafs belong all *equations*, or propofitions relating to number and quantity, that is, all that admit of mathematical demonftration, as *twice two is four, and the three angles of a right lined triangle are equal to two right angles*. For when the terms of thefe propofitions are duly confidered, it is found that they do not really differ, but exprefs the very fame quantity. This is, in its own nature, a conviction or perfuafion of the fulleft kind.

Thefe two kinds of propofitions, being very different in their natures, require very different kinds of *proof*.

The *evidence*, that any two things or properties are neceffarily united is the conftant obfervation of their union. It having always been obferved, for inftance, that the milk of animals is white, the idea of *white* becomes a neceffary part, or attendant of the idea of *milk*.

In other words, we call it an *eſſential property* of milk. This, however, only reſpects the milk of thoſe animals with which we are acquainted. But ſince the milk of all the animals with which we are acquainted, or of which we have heard, is white, we can have no reaſon to ſuſpect that the milk of any new and ſtrange animal is of any other colour. Alſo, ſince wherever there has been the ſpecific gravity, ductility, and other properties of *gold*, the colour has always been *yellow*, we conclude that thoſe circumſtances are neceſſarily united, though by ſome unknown bond of union, and that they will always go together.

The proper *proof*, therefore, of univerſal propoſitions, ſuch as the above, that milk is white, that gold is yellow, or that a certain degree of cold will freeze water, conſiſts in what is called an *induction of particular facts*, of preciſely the ſame nature. Having found, by much and various experience, that the ſame events never fail to take place in the ſame circumſtances,

ſtances; the *expectation* of the ſame conſequences from the ſame previous circumſtances is neceſſarily generated in our minds, and we can have no more ſuſpicion of a different event, than we can ſeparate the idea of *whiteneſs* from that of the other properties of *milk*.

Thus when the previous circumſtances are preciſely the ſame, we call the proceſs of proof by the name of *induction*. But if they be not preciſely the ſame, but only bear a conſiderable reſemblance to the circumſtances from which any particular appearance has been found to reſult, we call the argument *analogy*; and it is ſtronger in proportion to the degree of reſemblance in the previous circumſtances. Thus if we have found the milk of all the animals with which we are acquainted to be nouriſhing, though the natures of thoſe animals be conſiderably different, we think it probable that the milk of any ſtrange animal will be nouriſhing. If, therefore, the evidence of a propoſition of this kind be weak, or doubtful, it can be ſtrengthened only

only by finding more facts of the same, or of a similar nature.

If the truth of a proposition of the other class be not self evident, that is, if the subject and predicate do not appear, at first sight, to be different names for the same thing, another term must be found that shall be synonymous to them both. Thus, to prove that the three internal angles of a right lined triangle are equal to two right angles, I produce the base of the triangle; and having, by this means; made it evident that all the internal angles are equal to three angles formed by lines drawn from the same point in a right line, which I know to be equal to two right angles, the demonstration is complete.

This process exactly corresponds to the method of learning and teaching the signification of words in an unknown language, by means of one that is known. I may not know, for instance, what is meant by the Latin word *domus;* but if

I be

I be informed that it has the ſame meaning with *maiſon* in French, with which I am well acquainted, it immediately occurs to me, that it muſt have the ſame ſignification as *houſe* in Engliſh. And as the idea of a *houſe* was perfectly aſſociated with the word *maiſon*, I no ſooner put the word *domus* in its place, than the idea that was at firſt annexed to the word *maiſon* becomes connected with the word *domus*. For ſome time, however, the word *domus* will not excite the idea of a houſe without the help of the word *maiſon;* but by degrees it gets united to the idea immediately, ſo that afterwards they will be as inſeparable as the ſame idea and the word *maiſon* was before.

In like manner, when *ſyllogiſms* become familiar, the ſubject and predicate of the propoſition to be proved unite, and coaleſce immediately, without the help of the *middle term;* in which caſe the concluſion is as inſtantaneous as a ſimple judgment. In this manner it is that authority, as that of a parent, or of God, pro-

produces instant conviction. We first put confidence in them, and then the moment that any thing is known to have their sanction, it engages our assent and acquiescence.

I may see no natural connection, for instance, between this life and another: but firmly believing that the declarations of Jesus Christ have the sanction of divine authority, which I know cannot deceive me: the moment I find that he has asserted that there will be a resurrection of the dead to a future life, it becomes an article of my faith; and not the least perceivable space of time is lost in forming the two syllogisms, by which I conclude, first, that what Christ says is true, because he speaks by commission from God; and secondly, that the doctrine of the resurrection is true, because he has asserted it.

In fact, both *propositions* and *syllogisms* are things of *art* and not of *nature*. The ideas belonging to the two terms of of milk and whitenefs, out of which is formed the propofition *milk is white*, were originally impreffed, as was obferved before, at the fame time, and only formed a fingle complex idea. So alfo the moment that any two terms coalefce, as *lac* in Latin, and *milk* in Englifh, the ideas annexed to the word milk and that of whitenefs among the reft, are immedately transferred to the word *lac*, without any formal fyllogifm.

The word *truth*, and the idea annexed to it, is alfo the child of art, and not of nature, as well as the ideas annexed to the words *propofition* and *fyllogifm*. Ideas coalefce in our minds by the principle of affociation, thefe affociations extend themfelves, and ideas belonging to one word are transferred to another, without our giving any attention to thefe mental operations or affections. But when thefe proceffes have taken place in our minds many times, we are capable of obferving them, as well as the ideas which are the fubject of them; and we give names to

thefe

these mental processes just as we do to the affections of things without ourselves.

Thus the perfect *coincidence* of the ideas belonging to different terms, as *twice two* and *four*, and likewise the universal and necessary *concurrence* of two ideas, as those of *milk* and *whiteness*, having been observed, we make use of some term, *truth*, for instance, to express either of those circumstances; for being very much alike, it has not been found necessary to distinguish them by different appellations.

Since propositions and reasoning are mental operations, and, in fact, nothing more than cases of the *association of ideas*, every thing necessary to the processes may take place in the mind of a child, of an ideot, or of a brute animal, and produce the proper affections and actions, in proportion to the extent of their intellectual powers. The *knowledge of these operations*, which is gained by the attention we give to them, is a thing of a

very

very different nature, juſt as different as the knowledge of the nature of viſion is different from viſion itſelf. The philoſopher only is acquainted with the ſtructure of the eye, and the theory of viſion, but the clown ſees as well as he does, and makes as good uſe of his eyes.

Suppoſe a dog to have been puſhed into a fire, and ſeverely burned. Upon this, the idea of *fire* and the idea that has been left by the painful ſenſation of *burning* become intimately aſſociated together; ſo that the idea of being puſhed into the fire, and the idea of the pain that was the conſequence of it are ever after inſeparable. He cannot tell you in words, that *fire has a power of burning*, becauſe he has not the faculty of ſpeech; or, though he might have ſigns to expreſs *fire* and *burning*, he might not have got ſo abſtract an idea as that of *power;* but, notwithſtanding this, the two ideas of *fire* and of *burning* are as intimately united in his mind, as they can be in the mind of a philoſopher, who has reflected upon his

mental

mental affections, and is able to describe that union, or association of ideas, in proper terms.

If you endeavour to push the dog into the fire, he will instantly spring from it, before he has felt any thing of the heat; which as clearly shows his apprehension of danger from a situation in which he suffered before, as if he could have explained the foundation of his fear in the form of regular syllogisms and conclusions. No philosopher, who can analize the operations of his mind, and discourse concerning them, could reason more justly, more effectually, or more expeditiously, than he does.

*Words* are of great *use* in the business of thinking, but are not necessary to it. In like manner though the knowledge of *logic* is not without its use, it is by no means necessary for the purpose of reasoning. And as the doctrine of *syllogisms* was deduced from observations on reasoning, just as other *theories* are deduced

deduced from facts previously known; so the doctrine of *propositions* and *judgment* was deduced from observations on the coincidence of ideas, which took place antecedent to any knowledge of that kind.

There is hardly any thing to which we give the name of *opinion*, or *belief*, that does not require some degree of abstraction, and knowledge of what passes within the mind. And the common actions of life, which may be *analized* into opinions and reasoning, and which discover what we call sagacity in a very high degree, may be performed without any such thing, that is without any explicit knowledge of such mental affections and operations. Let us, for an example of this, take *the belief of an external world*. This is thought to be universal; and yet it appears to me to be very possible, not only that the lower animals, but even that children may not have reflected so much as that, properly speaking, they can be said to have formed any such opinion.

When ſenſation firſt takes place, the child has no notices of any thing but by means of certain impreſſions, generally called *ſenſations*, which objects excite in his mind, by means of the organs of ſenſe, and their correſponding nerves. Suppoſing the ſenſes to be perfect, and expoſed to the influence of external objects, the child is immediately ſenſible of theſe impreſſions; ſome of which give him pleaſure, others pain, and others ſenſations between both. At the ſame time the muſcular ſyſtem is peculiarly irritable, ſo that thoſe muſcles which are afterwards moſt perfectly ſubject to the voluntary power are almoſt continually in action, but in a random and automatic manner, as long as the child is awake and in health.

Let us ſuppoſe now that his own *hand* paſſes frequently before his eye. The impreſſion of it will be conveyed to the mind; and when, by any kind of mechaniſm (vibrations, or any thing elſe) that impreſſion is revived, he will get a fixed

fixed idea of his hand. Let now any painful impreſſion be made upon his hand, as by the flame of a candle. The violence that is thereby done to his nerves will throw the whole nervous and muſcular ſyſtem into agitation, and will more eſpecially occaſion the contraction of thoſe muſcles which are neceſſary to withdraw his hand from the object that gave him pain, as Dr. Hartley has ſhewn by curious anatomical diſquiſitions in a variety of inſtances. Admitting then the principle of the aſſociation of ideas; after a ſufficient number of theſe joint impreſſions, the action of drawing back his hand will mechanically follow the idea of the near approach of the candle.

In a manner equally mechanical, deſcribed at length by Dr. Hartley, the motions of *reaching* and *graſping* at things that give children pleaſure are acquired by them. And in time, by the ſame proceſs, the ideas of things that give us pleaſure or pain become aſſociated with a variety of other motions, beſides the mere

 withdrawing

withdrawing of the hand and thrusting it forward, &c. and these also, as well as many circumstances attending those states of mind get their own separate associations; so that, at length, a great variety of methods of pursuing pleasure and avoiding pain is acquired by us.

When the different impressions nearly balance one another, the ideas, or motions in the brain, interfering with and checking one another, some sensible space of time intervenes before the final determination to pursue any particular object, or to use any particular method of gaining the object takes place. To this state of mind, when we observe it, we give the name of *deliberation*, and to the determination itself, that of *will*. But still that motion, or connected train of motions, will take place which is the most intimately connected with, and dependent upon the state of mind, or impressions, immediately previous to it.

It

It will readily be concluded from this, that the more extenſive are the intellectual powers, that is, the greater is the number of ideas, and conſequently their aſſociations, the oftener will this caſe of *deliberation*, or *ſuſpence*, occur. Brutes are hardly ever at a loſs what to do, and children ſeldom; ſo that to explain their actions we have hardly any occaſion for the uſe of the terms *deliberation*, *volition*, or *will*; the ideas of every pleaſureable and painful object being immediately followed by one particular definite action, proper to ſecure the one and avoid the other; the tendencies to other actions having never interfered to check and retard it. Now it can only be during this ſtate of deliberation, and ſuſpence, that we have any opportunity of perceiving, and attending to what paſſes within our own minds; ſo that a conſiderable *compaſs of intellect*, a large ſtock of ideas, and much experience, are neceſſary to this reflection, and the knowledge that is gained by it.

We fee, then, that a child, or brute animal, is in poffeffion of a power of purfuing pleafure and avoiding pain, and, in like manner, a power of purfuing other intermediate and different objects, in confequence of impreffions made upon their minds by things external to them, without their having given any attention to the affections or operations of their minds; and indeed, confequently, without having fuch an idea as that of *mind* at all, or hardly of *felf*. Some brute animals may poffibly never advance farther than this; excepting that, their pleafurable and painful impreffions being affociated with a variety of particular perfons and circumftances, they will neceffarily acquire the rudiments of all the *paffions*, as of joy and forrow, love and hatred, gratitude and refentment, hope and fear, &c. each of which may be as *intenfe*, though lefs *complex* than they are found in the human fpecies. Indeed they will be more fenfible, and quick in their operations and effects, from the want of that variety of affociations which take place in our minds,

and

and which check and overrule one another.

It is evident, however, that if time and opportunity be given for the purpoſe, (which, for the reaſon aſſigned above, can only be obtained where there is a conſiderable compaſs of intellect, and much exerciſe of it) the *affections* of our ideas are as capable of being the ſubjects of obſervation as the *ideas* themſelves, juſt as the attractions, repulſions, and various affections of external bodies may be obſerved, as well as the bodies themſelves. And it is poſſible that, at length, no affection or modification of ideas ſhall take place, without leaving what we may call an *idea* of every part of the proceſs. And as we give names to other things which are diſtinguiſhed by certain properties, ſo we give the name of *mind, ſentient principle,* or *intellect,* to that within ourſelves in which theſe ideas exiſt, and theſe operations are performed.

At firſt a child can have no notion of any difference between external objects themſelves, and the immediate objects of his contemplation. He has no knowledge, for inſtance, of impreſſions being made by viſible things on his eye, and ſtill leſs has he any knowledge of the nerves or brain. But having given ſufficient attention to the phenomena of viſion, and of the other ſenſes, he is convinced, firſt, that the eye, the ear, or ſome other ſenſe is neceſſary to convey to him the knowledge of external objects; and that without theſe organs of ſenſe, he would have been for ever inſenſible of all that paſſed without himſelf.

By attending to theſe obſervations he is likewiſe convinced, that the immediate objects of his attention are not, as he before imagined, the *external things themſelves*, but ſome affection of his ſenſes, occaſioned by them. Afterwards he finds that his eye, his ear, and other organs of ſenſe, cannot convey to him the knowledge of any thing, unleſs there be a

communication

communication between theſe organs and the brain, by means of proper *nerves*; which convinces him that the immediate objects of his thoughts are not in the organs of ſenſe, but in the *brain*, farther than which he is not able to trace any thing.

This kind of knowledge is gained by obſervation and experiment, as much as the theory of the eye and of light, though we ourſelves are the ſubject of the obſervations and experiments. And our thinking and acting, in the conduct of life, is as much independent of this branch of knowledge, as the powers of air and light are independent of our knowledge of them.

Having, by this proceſs, gained the knowledge of the diſtinction between the immediate objects of our thoughts, and external objects, it may occur to ſome perſons, that, ſince we are not properly *conſcious*, or *know in the firſt inſtance*, any thing more than what paſſes within ourſelves,

ourſelves, that is, our own ſenſations and ideas, theſe may be impreſſed upon the mind without the help of any thing external to us, by the immediate agency of the author of our being. This no philoſopher will ſay is impoſſible, but, of two hypotheſes to account for the ſame phenomenon, he will conſider which is the more probable, as being more conſonant to the courſe of nature in other reſpects.

Half the inhabitants of the globe, for inſtance, may be looking towards the heavens at the ſame time, and all their minds are impreſſed in the ſame manner. All ſee the moon, ſtars, and planets, in preciſely the ſame ſituations; and even the obſervations of thoſe who uſe teleſcopes correſpond with the utmoſt exactneſs. To explain this, Biſhop Berkley ſays, that the divine being, attending to each individual mind, impreſſes their ſenſoriums in the ſame, or a correſponding manner, without the medium of any thing external to them. On the other hand,

hand, another perſon, without pretending that his ſcheme is impoſſible, where divine power is concerned, may think, however, that it is more natural to ſuppoſe that there really *are* ſuch bodies as the moon, ſtars, and planets, placed at certain diſtances from us, and moving in certain directions; by means of which, and a more general agency of the deity than Biſhop Berkley ſuppoſes, all our minds are neceſſarily impreſſed in this correſponding manner.

It is ſufficient evidence for this hypotheſis, that it exhibits *particular appearances*, as ariſing from *general laws*, which is agreeable to the analogy of every thing elſe that we obſerve. It is recommended by the ſame *ſimplicity* that recommends every other philoſophical theory, and needs no other evidence whatever; and I ſhould think that a perſon muſt have very little knowledge of the nature of *philoſophy*, who ſhould think of having recourſe to any other for the purpoſe. Dr. Reid, however, not ſatisfied with this evidence,

evidence, pretends that the certain belief of the real exiſtence of external objects is arbitrarily connected with the ideas of them. The hypotheſis of *knowing things by means of ideas only,* he ſays, 'Dedi-'cation,' p. 7, 'is antient, indeed, and has 'been generally received by philoſophers, 'but of which I could find no ſolid proof. 'The hypotheſis I mean is, that nothing 'is perceived but what is in the mind 'which perceives it: That we do not 'really perceive things that are external, 'but only certain images and pictures of 'them, imprinted upon the mind, which 'are called *impreſſions* and *ideas.*'

In fact, it is not true that we neceſſarily believe the exiſtence of external objects, *as diſtinct from our ideas of them.* Originally, we have no knowledge of any ſuch thing as *ideas,* any more than we have of the images of objects on the retina; and the moment we have attained to the knowledge of ideas, the external world is nothing more than an *hypotheſis,* to account for thoſe ideas; ſo probable, in-

deed,

deed, that few perſons ſeriouſly doubt of its real exiſtence, and of its being the cauſe of our ideas. But ſtill the contrary may be affirmed without any proper *abſurdity*. Thus, alſo, the revolution of the planets round the ſun beſt accounts for the appearances of nature, but the contrary may be ſuppoſed and affirmed without ſubjecting a perſon to the charge of talking *nonſenſe*. This, however, is the language that is now adopted when any of the dictates of a pretended principle of *common ſenſe* is controverted; and one of the arbitrary decrees of this new infallible guide to truth is, it ſeems, the reality of an external world.

Such is the leading principle of that philoſophy which I principally mean to combat in the enſuing Remarks on the writings of Dr. Reid, Dr. Beattie, and Dr. Oſwald.

# REMARKS

ON

# Dr. REID's INQUIRY

INTO THE

# PRINCIPLES

OF THE

# HUMAN MIND.

THE

# INTRODUCTION.

THE great businefs of philofophy is to reduce into claffes the various appearances which nature prefents to our view. For by this means we acquire an eafy and diftinct knowledge of them, and gain a more perfect comprehenfion of their various natures, relations, and ufes. Nature prefents to our view *particular effects*, in connection with their *feparate caufes*, by which we are often puzzled, till philofophy fteps in to our affiftance, pointing out a fimilarity in thefe effects, and the probability of fuch fimilar effects arifing from the fame caufe. Having got into this track of *fimplifying* all appearances, and all caufes, we are able to predict new appearances from their known previous circumftances; and thus we add to our own power, convenience, and happineſs, by availing ourſelves of the powers of nature.

A very conſiderable advance has been made in this truly philoſophical and uſeful progreſs with reſpect to the knowledge of the world around us, and the laws by which it is governed. And the knowledge of *ourſelves*, both body and mind, has likewiſe advanced in the proportion that might have been expected from the natural order of our thoughts; which are firſt engaged by an attention to external objects before we reflect upon ourſelves. Something was done in this field of knowledge by Deſcartes, very much by Mr. Locke, but moſt of all by Dr. Hartley, who has thrown more uſeful light upon the theory of the mind than Newton did upon the theory of the natural world.

But while ſome are employed in making real advances in the knowledge of nature, there have always been others poſſeſſed not always, perhaps, of envious but of little and contracted minds, who, instead of doing, or attempting to do any thing themselves, are busily employed in watching the footsteps of others, and cavilling at every thing they do; which is not without a good effect, as it obliges philosophers to use greater caution and circumspection, to review their steps, and tread upon surer ground than they would otherwise do.

Every discovery in natural philosophy made by Copernicus, Galileo, or Newton, was disputed inch by inch; and can we be surprised that the labours of Mr. Locke should share the same fate? As to Dr. Hartley, his *day of trial* is not yet come, and one of my views in this publication, and some others that I have projected, is to bring it on; not doubting but that it will stand the test, and be better known, and more firmly established after such a scrutiny.

The fate of Mr. Locke's principles of the human mind has, however, been rather ſingularly hard. The ſyſtems of other philoſophers, after having been fully and rigorouſly criticized, have generally been acquieſced in; but his, after having undergone this ſtrict examination from all the learned of his own age, and having been acquieſced in for near a century, has met with a more rude, and more pertinacious ſet of adverſaries; who inſtead of allowing the knowledge of the mind to advance with the knowledge of nature in general, appear to me to be throwing every thing into its priſtine confuſion, and even introducing more darkneſs than naturally ever belonged to the ſubject.

The outlines of Mr. Locke's ſyſtem are, that the mind perceives all things that are external to it by means of certain impreſſions, made upon the organs of ſenſe; that thoſe impreſſions are conveyed by the nerves to the brain, and from the brain to the mind, where they are called *ſenſations,* and when recollected are called *ideas;* that by the attention which the mind, or ſentient principle, gives to theſe

ſenſations

ſenſations and ideas, obſerving their mutual relations, *&c.* it acquires other ideas, which he calls *ideas of reflection*, and thereby becomes poſſeſſed of the materials of all its knowledge. Other things he has adopted, and taken for granted concerning the mind, which are not well founded; and I think he has been haſty in concluding that there is ſome other ſource of our ideas beſides the external ſenſes; but the reſt of his ſyſtem appears to me, and others, to be the corner ſtone of all juſt and rational knowledge of ourſelves.

This ſolid foundation, however, has lately been attempted to be overturned by a ſet of pretended philoſophers, of whom the moſt conſpicuous and aſſuming is Dr. Reid, profeſſor of moral philoſophy in the univerſity of Glaſgow, who, in order to combat Biſhop Berkley, and the ſcepticiſm of Mr. Hume, has himſelf introduced almoſt univerſal ſcepticiſm and confuſion; denying all the connections which had before been ſuppoſed to ſubſiſt between the ſeveral phænomena, powers, and operations of the mind, and ſubſtituting ſuch a number of *independent, arbitrary, inſtinctive principles*, that the very enumeration of them is really tireſome.

It is very poſſible, indeed, and no perſon can deny it, that we may proceed too rapidly in ſimplifying appearances, and therefore ſuch writers as Dr. Reid are an uſeful and ſeaſonable check upon us. But, on the other hand, ſo looſe and incoherent a ſyſtem as he would ſubſtitute in the place of Mr. Locke's, ought not to be adopted without the moſt urgent neceſſity; ſince it wants the recommendation of that agreeable *ſimplicity*, which is ſo apparent in other parts of the conſtitution of nature. Appearances and analogy being ſo much againſt this ſyſtem, we are juſtified in requiring the ſtronger evidence for it.

It is impoſſible to contemplate ſuch a theory of the human mind as that of Dr. Reid

Reid with any ſatisfaction, and the farther ſtudy of the ſubject is thereby rendered exceedingly diſguſting and unpromiſing. I flatter myſelf therefore, that I may be doing ſome ſervice to future inquirers, by endeavouring to ſhow that this new ſyſtem has in it as little of truth, as it has of beauty, that we may ſafely take up the ſubject, where Mr. Locke left it, and proceed to attend to what Dr. Hartley has done by following his ſteps; when, if I have any foreſight, we ſhall ſmile at Dr. Reid's hypotheſis, or rather ſtring of hypotheſes as a mere puzzle, and look back upon it as upon a dream.

To proceed with as much perſpicuity as I poſſibly can in this perplexed ſubject, I ſhall firſt preſent my reader with a view of all the unconnected inſtinctive principles which Dr. Reid pretends to have diſcovered in the mind, and I ſhall then examine, in diſtinct ſections, his objections to Mr. Locke's doctrine, and the foundation he has laid for his own peculiar hypotheſes.

That I may preſerve at the ſame time the greateſt diſtinctneſs with reſpect to my reader, and the greateſt fairneſs with reſpect to the author on whom I am animadverting, I ſhall enumerate all the pretended inſtinctive principles of which he has given any account in this treatiſe, and exhibit them in the form of a *table*, ſubjoining my authorities, in quotations from thoſe different parts of his work from which I have collected them, and alſo numbering the articles, ſo that they may correſpond to one another, and be eaſily compared together.

# SECTION I.

## *A Table of Dr.* Reid's *inſtinctive principles.*

| | | | |
|---|---|---|---|
| 1 | A preſent ſenſation ſuggeſts | | the belief of the preſent exiſtence of an object. |
| | Memory | —— | the belief of its paſt exiſtence. |
| | Imagination | —— | no belief at all. |
| 2 | Mental affections | —— | the idea and belief of our own exiſtence. |
| 3 | Odours, taſtes, ſounds, and certain affections of the optic nerve | —— | their peculiar correſponding ſenſations. |
| 4 | A hard ſubſtance | —— | the ſenſation of hardneſs, and the belief of ſomething hard. |
| 5 | An extended ſubſtance | — | the idea of extenſion and ſpace. |
| 6 | All the primary qualities of bodies | —— | their peculiar ſenſations. |
| 5 | A body in motion | —— | the idea of motion. |
| 6 | Certain forms of the features, articulations of the voice, and attitudes of the body | —— | the idea and belief of certain thoughts, purpoſes, and diſpoſitions of the mind. |
| 7 | Inverted images on the retina | —— | upright viſion. |
| 8 | Images in correſponding parts of both eyes*. | —— | ſingle viſion |
| 9 | Pains in any part of the body | —— | the idea of the place where the pain is ſeated. |

*He alſo enumerates the following among inſtinctive faculties or principles,* viz.

10 The parallel motion of the eyes, as neceſſary to diſtinct viſion.
11 The ſenſe of veracity, or a diſpoſition to ſpeak truth.
12 A ſenſe of credulity, or a diſpoſition to believe others.
12 The inductive faculty, by which we infer ſimilar effects from ſimilar cauſes.

*N. B.* All theſe ſeparate inſtinctive principles Dr. Reid conſiders as branches of what he terms *common ſenſe*.

* Different animals are ſubject to different laws in this reſpect.

*Authorities*

*Authorities for the preceding table.*

1. 'SENSATION compels our belief 'of the present existence of a 'thing, memory the belief of its past 'existence, and imagination no belief at 'all. These are all simple and original, 'and therefore inexplicable acts of the 'mind.' p. 31.

'The connexion between our sensa-'tions and the conception and belief of 'external existences cannot be produced 'by habit, education, or any principle of 'human nature that has been admitted 'by philosophers.' p. 91.

'A third class of natural signs compre-'hends those which, tho' we never be-'fore had any notion or conception of 'the things signified, do suggest it, or 'conjure it up, as it were, by a natural 'kind of magic, and at once give us a 'conception, and create a belief of it. 'p. 90. This class of natural signs is the 'foundation

'foundation of *common sense*, a part of 'human nature which has never been 'explained.' p. 91.

'Sensation, and the perception of ex-'ternal objects by the senses, tho' very 'different in their nature, have commonly 'been considered as one and the same 'thing.' p. 288.

'I know that the perception of an 'object implies both the conception of 'its form, and a belief of its present ex-'istence. I know, moreover, that this 'belief is not the effect of argument and 'reasoning. It is the immediate effect 'of my constitution.' p. 290.

2. 'The idea of our own existence 'precedes all reasoning and experience.' p. 48.

3. See p. 84, quoted below, and his treatise passim.

4. By an original principle of our
'constitution a certain sensation of touch 'both suggests to the mind the conception of hardness, and creates the belief of it, or in other words, this sensation is a natural sign of hardness.' p. 86.

5. 'Space, motion, and extension, 'and all the primary qualities of bodies, 'have no resemblance to any sensation or 'any operation of our minds, and therefore cannot be ideas either of sensation 'or reflection. The very conception of 'them is irreconcileable to the principles 'of all our philosophical systems of the 'universe. The belief of them is no less 'so.' p. 102.

'The notion of extension is so familiar 'to us from our infancy, and so constantly obtruded by every thing we see 'or feel, that we are apt to think it obvious how it comes into the mind; but 'upon a narrower examination we shall 'find it utterly inexplicable. It is true 'we 'we have feelings of touch, which every 'moment present extension to the mind; 'but how they come to do so is the que'stion: for those feelings do no more re'semble extension than they resemble 'justice or courage, nor can the existence 'of extended things be inferred from 'those feelings by any rule of reasoning; 'so that the feelings we have by touch 'can neither explain how we get the no'tion, nor how we come by the belief of 'extended things.' p. 96.

6. 'The thoughts, purposes, and dis'positions of the mind, have their na'tural signs in the features of the face, 'the modification of the voice, and the 'attitude of the body. p. 87. In these 'natural signs,' he says, ib. 'there is, as 'in artificial signs, often neither simili'tude between the sign and the thing 'signified, nor any connection that arises 'necessarily from the nature of things.' Of these particular natural signs he says, p. 89, that 'they are not only esta'blished by nature, but discovered to us

'by

'by a natural principle, without reaſon-
'ing or experience. An infant, he adds,
'may be put in a fright by an angry
'countenance, and ſoothed again by
'ſigns and blandiſhments.'

7. See ch. i. ſection xi. paſſim.

8. 'The correſpondence of certain 'points in the retinæ is prior to the 'habits we acquire in viſion, and conſe- 'quently is natural and original.' p. 261.

'Since there is a prodigious variety 'in the ſtructure, the motions, and the 'number of eyes in different animals and 'inſects, it is probable that the laws 'by which viſion is regulated are not 'the ſame in all, but various, adapted to 'the eyes which nature has given them.' p. 233. See alſo ch. vi. ſection xiii. paſſim.

9. 'How do we know the parts of our body affected by particular pains?

'not

'not by experience, or by reaſoning, but 'by the conſtitution of nature.' p. 209.

10. 'The parallel motion of the eyes 'we reſolve into an original power and 'principle of the human mind, and not 'to be referred to cuſtom, to anatomical 'or mechanical cauſes.' p. 185. He alſo calls it a *natural inſtinct*, p. 187. But ſee ch. vi. ſection x. paſſim.

11. 'There is in the human mind an 'early anticipation, neither derived from 'experience nor reaſoning, nor from any 'compact or promiſe, that our fellow-'creatures will uſe the ſame ſigns in lan-'guage when they have the ſame ſenti-'ments. This is, in reality, a kind of 'preſcience of human actions, and ſeems 'to me to be an original principle of the 'human conſtitution, without which we 'ſhould be incapable of language, and 'conſequently incapable of inſtruction.' p. 336.

'The wiſe author of our nature has 'implanted in our natures two prin- 'ciples that tally with each other, the 'firſt is a propenſity to ſpeak truth, and 'to uſe the ſigns of language ſo as to 'convey our real ſentiments, p. 336. 'Another original principle implanted 'in us by the ſupreme being, is a diſpo- 'ſition to confide in the veracity of 'others, and to believe what they tell 'us. This is the counterpart to the 'former; and as that may be called *the 'principle of veracity*, we ſhall, for want 'of a more proper name, call this *the 'principle of credulity*.'

12. 'The belief of the continuance 'of the preſent courſe of nature muſt be 'the effect of inſtinct, and not of reaſon, 'p. 343. All our knowledge of nature 'beyond our original perceptions is got 'by experience, and conſiſts in the in- 'terpretation of natural ſigns. The ap- 'pearance of the ſign is followed by the 'belief of the thing ſignified. Upon this 'principle of our conſtitution not only

'acquired

'acquired perception, but alſo inductive 'reaſoning, and all our reaſoning from 'analogy is grounded; and therefore, 'for want of another name, we ſhall beg 'leave to call it the *inductive principle*. 'It is from the force of this principle that 'we immediately aſſent to that axiom, 'upon which all our knowledge of nature 'is built, that effects of the ſame kind 'muſt have the ſame cauſe, p. 347. 'Take away the light of this inductive 'principle, and experience is as blind as 'a mole. She may indeed feel what is 'preſent, and what immediately touches 'her; but ſhe ſees nothing that is either 'before or behind, upon the right hand 'or upon the left, future or paſt.' p. 349.

It will be obſerved, that in this table I have connected the name of the thing or circumſtance that gives riſe to the correſponding feeling by the word *ſuggeſt*. This, however, is not to be miſtaken for a mere form of connection. Our author would have us to conſider it in a much more ſerious light, as a real power of the

 mind,

mind, which had escaped the notice of all the philosophers who had gone before him in these researches. '*Suggestion,*' he says, p. 49. 'is a power of the mind 'which seems entirely to have escaped 'the notice of philosophers, and to which 'we owe many of our simple notions 'which are neither impressions nor ideas, 'as well as many original principles of 'belief.

My reader will, I suspect, imagine with me, that this catalogue of original instinctive principles is pretty large, and that when nature had gone so far in this track, but little could be wanting to accomplish all her purposes; and that, with respect to *principles,* little remained to be done by any other means. But our author, it seems, thinks differently. 'The 'original perceptions which nature gives 'are insufficient,' he says, p. 351, 'for 'the purposes of life, and therefore she has 'made men capable of acquiring many 'more perceptions by habit.' Now my view in the following inquiry is to relieve

dame

dame nature of the unneceſſary load which Dr. Reid has laid upon her, by aſcribing a little more to habit, and to the neceſſary connections and conſequences of things than he has done.

When my reader ſhall have given ſufficient attention to the preceding table, and the authorities from which it was collected, I hope that he, our author, and myſelf, may proceed with a perfectly right underſtanding of one another. However, to complete this good underſtanding, and to prevent the poſſibility of a miſtake, I ſhall ſubjoin a few more extracts, which ſhow how perfectly independent of one another Dr. Reid imagined the principles enumerated in this table to be.

'No man can give a reaſon why the 'vibration of a body might not have 'given the ſenſation of ſmelling, and the 'effluvia of bodies affected our hearing, 'if it had ſo pleaſed our maker. In like 'manner no man can give a reaſon why 'the ſenſations of ſmell or taſte might 'not have indicated hardneſs, as well as 'that ſenſation which by our conſtitution 'does indicate it. Indeed no man can 'conceive any ſenſation to reſemble any 'known quality of bodies, nor can any 'man ſhow by any good argument that 'all our ſenſations might not have been 'as they are, tho' no body, or quality of 'bodies, had ever exiſted.' p. 84.

'Perhaps we might have been ſo made 'as to taſte with our fingers, to ſmell with 'our ears, and to hear by the noſe. Per'haps we might have been ſo made as to 'have all the perceptions and ſenſations 'which we have without any impreſſion 'made upon our bodily organs at all.' p. 305.

'The perceptions we have might have 'been immediately connected with the 'impreſſions of our organs, without any 'intervention of ſenſation. This laſt 'ſeems really to be the caſe in one in'ſtance, to wit, in our perception of the 'viſible figure of bodies.' p. 305.

'We

'We know nothing of the machinery 'by means of which every different im'preſſion upon the organs, nerves, and 'brain exhibits its correſponding ſenſa'tion, or of the machinery by means of 'which each ſenſation exhibits its corre'ſponding perception. We are inſpired 'with the ſenſation, and we are inſpired 'with the correſponding perception by 'means unknown.' p. 306.

Our author ſeems, however, to be willing to provide a decent retreat from his doctrine of original inſtinctive principles, by ſaying, p. 223, 'If in any caſe 'we ſhould give the name of a law of na'ture to a general phænomenon, which 'human induſtry ſhould afterwards trace 'to one more general, there is no great 'harm done. The moſt general aſſumes 'the name of a law of nature when it is 'diſcovered, and the leſs general is con'tained and comprehended in it.'

But I muſt take the liberty to ſay, that if this ſhould happen, harm *will* be done to the hypothesis of that man who had been so rash and unguarded as to advance over and over, so that no body could mistake his meaning, that a certain law of nature was absolutely *ultimate*, which afterwards appeared not to be so; who should have asserted that these principles are *simple, original*, and therefore *inexplicable acts of the mind*, and that they *cannot* be produced by any principle of human nature that has ever been admitted by philosophers. This is asserting that it is impossible to advance any farther in the investigation, for who can ever get beyond *simple, original*, and *inexplicable acts of the mind*.

The suspicion that we are got to ultimate principles necessarily checks all farther inquiry, and is therefore of great disservice in philosophy. Let Dr. Reid lay his hand upon his breast, and say, whether, after what he has written, he would not be exceedingly mortified to find it clearly proved, to the satisfaction of all the world, that all the instinctive princi-

ples

ples in the preceding table were really acquired, and that all of them were nothing more than ſo many different caſes of the old and well known principle of *aſſociation of ideas*.

It muſt, moreover, be obſerved, that the table I have given by no means contains a view of *all* the original inſtinctive principles which our ſagacious author finds in human nature. Theſe are only ſuch as have occurred to him in his ſurvey of the external ſenſes. 'We have 'taken notice,' he ſays, p. 378, 'of ſeveral 'original principles of belief in the courſe 'of this inquiry; and when other faculties 'of the mind are examined, we ſhall find 'more which have not occured in the 'examination of the five ſenſes.'

It may be ſaid that, ſince our author has not finiſhed his ſcheme, this critique upon it is premature, that we ought firſt to hear him out, and that it is not good manners to riſe from the table after the firſt courſe though we be not diſpoſed to partake of the ſecond. I anſwer, that Dr. Reid's gueſts have already waited about ten years, and that poſſibly this account of the firſt courſe may induce our hoſt to haſten his ſecond. To drop all figure: our author's ſcheme appears to be already complete as far as it goes, and the evidence of what is before us is altogether independent of what is to come; at leaſt there is no hint given to us of the contrary.

SEC-

## SECTION II.

*A view of the ſeveral fallacies by which* Dr. Reid *has been miſled in his inquiry.*

I Now proceed to conſider Dr. Reid's objections to the great outlines of Mr. Locke's doctrine, and the ſeveral principles on which he has founded his own; endeavouring, at the ſame time, to ſhew the ſufficiency of the commonly received principles for thoſe purpoſes for which Dr. Reid pretends that they are altogether inſufficient, ſo as to oblige him to quit them for others of his own.

As my remarks on the Doctor's performance were made in the courſe of reading him, and thereby things of a different nature will be unavoidably a little intermixed (though I ſhall take all the care I can in the arrangement of them) I ſhall introduce them with diſtinctly noting the ſeveral falſe ſteps which he has made in the courſe of it, or the different *fallacies* to which

which he ſeems to have been ſubject, and which have been the ſource of the principal of his miſtakes.

1. Becauſe he cannot perceive any reſemblance between objects and ideas, he concludes, that the one cannot be produced by the other.

2. Becauſe he cannot perceive any neceſſary connection between ſenſations and the objects of them, and therefore cannot abſolutely demonſtrate the reality of external objects, or even the exiſtence of mind itſelf, by the doctrine of ideas, he rejects that doctrine altogether, and has recourſe to arbitrary inſtincts.

3. He takes it for granted that our ideas have no exiſtence but when we are conſcious of them, and attend to them.

4. He confounds the faculty of ſenſation with ideas of ſenſation.

5. Becauſe we do not know the mechaniſm by which a particular motion, or a ſet

a ſet of connected motions, is performed, he concludes that thoſe motions are performed by inſtinctive principles, and were not acquired by experience and the aſſociation of ideas.

6. Suppoſing, without any foundation, that certain determinations or emotions were prior to experience, he concludes that they are inſtinctive.

Let it be noted, that I do not aſſert that our learned profeſſor is *uniform* in theſe miſtakes, for by ſome of my remarks I think it will appear that he is not perfectly conſiſtent with himſelf.

## SECTION III.

*Of Dr.* Reid's *objection to the doctrine of ideas from their want of resemblance to their corresponding objects.*

DR. Reid objects to every ſyſtem which ſuppoſes that the mind receives images of things from without by means of the ſenſes, and thinks that they are ſufficiently refuted by the obſervation, that ſenſations bear no reſemblance to bodies, or any of their qualities. ' The properties of extenſion, ' figure, ſolidity, motion, hardneſs, rough- ' neſs, as well as colour, heat, and cold, ' ſound, taſte, and ſmell, which all man- ' kind have conceived to be the qualities ' of bodies, have not', he ſays, p. 147, ' among them all, one ſingle image of ' body, or any of its qualities. I am ſure ' that, by proper attention and care, ' I may know my ſenſations, and be ' able to affirm with certainty what they ' reſemble, and what they do not reſem- ' ble.

'ble. I have examined them one by one, 'and compared them with matter and its 'qualities, and I cannot find one of them 'that confeſſes a reſembling feature.'

So very confident is our author of the ſtrength of this argument, that he ſcruples not to reſt the whole of his ſyſtem upon it. 'This,' ſays he, p. 108, 'I would 'humbly propoſe as an *experimentum* '*crucis*, by which the ideal ſyſtem muſt 'ſtand or fall; and it brings the matter 'to a ſhort iſſue. Extenſion, figure, mo-'tion, may, any one, or all of them, be 'taken for the ſubject of this experiment. 'Either they are ideas of ſenſation, or 'they are not. If any one of them can 'be ſhown to be an idea of ſenſation, or 'to have the leaſt reſemblance to any ſen-'ſation, I lay my hand upon my mouth, 'and give up all pretenſe to reconcile rea-'ſon to common ſenſe in this matter, and 'muſt ſuffer the ideal ſcepticiſm to tri-'umph. But if, on the other hand, they 'are not ideas of ſenſation, nor like to 'any ſenſation, then the ideal ſyſtem is a

'rope of ſand, and all the laboured argu-
'ments of the ſceptical philoſophy againſt
'a material world, and againſt the exi-
'ſtence of every thing but impreſſions
'and ideas, proceed upon a falſe hypo-
'theſis.'

Before our author had reſted ſo much upon this argument, it behoved him, I think, to have examined the ſtrength of it a little more carefully than he ſeems to have done; for he appears to me to have ſuffered himſelf to be miſled in the very foundation of it, merely by philoſophers happening to call ideas the *images* of external things; as if this was not known to be a figurative expreſſion, denoting not that the actual ſhapes of things were delineated in the brain, or upon the mind, but only that impreſſions of ſome kind or other were conveyed to the mind by means of the organs of ſenſe and their correſponding nerves, and that between theſe impreſſions and the ſenſations exiſting in the mind there is a real and neceſſary, though at preſent an unknown connection.

I do

I do not ſee but that by Dr. Reid's mode of reaſoning, he might as well deny that the ſound of a muſical ſtring is cauſed by the ſtroke of a *plectrum*, or that ſounds, conſidered as tremulous motions of the particles of the air, are produced by bodies ſtriking againſt one another, becauſe he can perceive no proper *reſemblance* between the cauſe and the effect, between the ſound that is produced and the ſhape of the thing or things by which the ſounds are made; and yet theſe ſounds vary according to the bodies that occaſion them, and the circumſtances that attend their impinging on one another; ſo that, without any ſuch reſemblance as the Doctor ſeems to expect, they correſpond ſtrictly to one another, and the one may be called the proper and *neceſſary*, and not the *arbitrary* (or as Dr. Reid would call it the *natural*) ſign of the other.

The transferring of this compariſon to the doctrine of ideas is very eaſy. If, as Dr. Hartley ſuppoſes, the nerves and brain be a vibrating ſubſtance, the analogy

logy will hold very nearly indeed; all ſenſations and ideas being vibrations in that ſubſtance, and all that is properly unknown in the buſineſs being the ſimple power in the mind to perceive, or be affected by, thoſe vibrations. And if, as Locke and others ſuppoſe, matter itſelf may be indued with that ſentient power, even that difficulty, as far as the preſent queſtion can be affected, is removed.

Our author's doubts are not confined to ideas being produced by external objects, but affect the uſe of the nerves belonging to the organs of ſenſe, and the brain itſelf, as the inſtruments of tranſmitting them to the mind, reducing the ſuppoſition to a mere probability.

'It is very probable,' he ſays, p. 200, 'that the optic nerve is the inſtrument of 'viſion, no leſs neceſſary than the retina.' But it appears to me that, arguing in this manner, one might doubt of every thing; and that we might juſt as well ſay it is very *probable* only that the feet and legs are

are the inſtruments of walking, as that the optic nerve is only *probably* the inſtrument of viſion.

In another place, he does not leave room to ſuppoſe that it is even probable that the optic nerves are the inſtrument of viſion; calling the hypotheſis a mere conjecture. 'From the firſt dawn of philoſophy to this day,' he ſays, p. 277, 'it has been believed that the optic nerves 'are intended to carry the images * of 'viſible objects from the bottom of the 'eye to the mind, and that the nerves be'longing to the other ſenſes have a like 'office. But how do we know this? We 'conjecture it, and taking this conjecture 'for a truth, we conſider how the nerves 'may beſt anſwer the purpoſe.' It is agreeable to this that he ſays, p. 303, 'We are inſpired with the ſenſation, and

* If Dr. Reid thinks to reconcile theſe two paſſages by ſaying that by *images*, in this place, he did not mean *impreſſions* in general, but the real *ſhapes* and *forms* of thing, the whole charge is falſe, and he is fighting a chimera of his own creating.

'we are inſpired with the correſponding
'perception, by means unknown.'

This ſcepticiſm with reſpect to the doctrine of ideas, the uſe of the organs of ſenſe, and their correſponding nerves in tranſmitting them, appears to me to be very extraordinary indeed; and yet, ſuch are the caprices of the human mind, Dr. Reid expreſſes as much ſurprize at the prevalence of the common opinion. 'It
'is very ſtrange,' he ſays, p. 201, 'that
'philoſophers of all ages ſhould have
'agreed in this notion, that the images
'of external objects are conveyed by the
'organs of ſenſe to the brain, and are
'there perceived by the mind. Nothing
'can be more unphiloſophical. For firſt
'this notion has no foundation in fact
'and obſervation. Of all the organs of
'ſenſe the eye only, as far as we can diſ-
'cover, forms any kind of image of its ob-
'ject, and the images formed by the eye
'are not in the brain, but only in the bot-
'tom of the eye; nor are they at all per-
'ceived or felt by the mind. Secondly,
'it

'it is as difficult to conceive how the 'mind perceives images in the brain, as 'how it perceives things more diſtant. If 'any man will ſhew how the mind may 'perceive images in the brain, I will un-'dertake to ſhew how it may perceive 'the moſt diſtant objects: for if we give 'eyes to the mind, to perceive what is 'tranſacted at home in its dark chamber, 'why may we not make theſe eyes a little 'longer ſighted, and then we ſhall have 'no occaſion for that unphiloſophical fic-'tion of images in the brain. In a word, 'the manner and mechaniſm of the mind's 'perception is quite beyond our compre-'henſion.'

In this way of arguing we might ſay that the whole ſyſtem of our ſenſes, nerves, and brain is of no real uſe whatever; for it is impoſſible to ſay *how* they act upon the mind, or the mind upon them. But by the ſame reaſoning we may deny every principle in nature. For when we have traced it as far as we can, we are ſtill compelled to ſtop ſomewhere, and to con-feſs our inability to proceed any farther.

I know, however, very well, that an eye is the inſtrument of viſion, becauſe without it nothing can be ſeen. I alſo know that the retina and optic nerve are likewiſe neceſſary, becauſe if they be diſordered, viſion is ſtill wanting; and laſtly, I am equally certain that the brain is neceſſary to all perception, becauſe if that be diſordered, thinking either intirely ceaſes, or is proportionably diſturbed.

For my part, I know no concluſions in philoſophy more certain than theſe, and they are not rendered at all leſs certain by our not being able to go a ſtep farther, ſo as to know in what *manner* the brain, or the affections of it, can be the inſtrument or ſubject of perception. I may conjecture that the brain itſelf may be the ultimate cauſe, or I may ſubſtitute ſomething elſe that I may think better adapted to anſwer the purpoſe, that is, to ſuit the phenomena.

## SECTION IV.

*Of Dr.* Reid's *objection to Mr.* Locke's *division of ideas into those of sensation and reflection.*

HAVING examined one great pillar of our author's scheme, I now proceed to another, of which he likewise boasts great things; but if my reader be able to consider it with perfect seriousness, it is more than I can expect of him, for it is more than I am able to do myself. It is his objection to Mr. Locke's division of ideas into those of *sensation*, and those of *reflection.*

'This', he says, p. 575, 'is contrary to 'all rules of logic, because the second 'member of the division includes the 'first. For can we form clear and just 'notions of our sensations any other way 'than by reflection? Surely we cannot. 'Sensation is an operation of the mind, of 'which we are conscious, and we get the 'notion of ſenſation by reflecting upon 'that which we are conſcious of. In like 'manner doubting and believing are 'operations of the mind, whereof we are 'conſcious, and we get the notion of 'them by reflecting upon what we are 'conſcious. The ideas of ſenſation there-'fore, are ideas of reflection, as much as 'the ideas of doubting or believing, or 'any other idea whatſoever.'

This I ſcruple not to ſay is as mere a quibble, as either the ignorance or the perverſion of logic ever produced, ariſing from our author's confounding the proper *ideas of ſenſation* with the idea of *ſenſation itſelf*, which is, no doubt, of the ſame claſs with the ideas of *doubting*, *believing*, or thoſe of any other operation of the mind; and ſo Mr. Locke would have acknowledged. But the ideas belonging to the claſs of ſenſation do not require any ſcientifical knowledge of that power, or any reflection upon it. If this were the caſe, brute animals, having no proper ideas of reflection, could have no ideas of ſenſation.

ſenſation. Indeed, it is queſtionable whether the bulk of mankind, who are not philoſophers, could have them, and conſequently whether they muſt not be deſtitute of all ideas.

A more palpable blunder than this I think I hardly ever met with in any argumentative treatiſe, and yet this is one of the great engines with which our author aſſails Mr. Locke's doctrine of ideas. Dr. Reid might juſt as well ſay that *houſes* and *utenſils* neceſſarily belong to the ſame claſs of objects, and that they ought never to be diſtinguiſhed, becauſe the former contain the latter.

Beſides our author himſelf ſuppoſes that even human beings may have ideas of mere ſenſation ſome time before they diſcover any power of reflection, and that this power may diſcover itſelf and come into play afterwards. 'Perhaps,' ſays he, p. 112, 'a child in the womb, or for 'ſome ſhort period of his exiſtence, is 'merely a ſentient being, the faculty by 'which it perceives an external world, 'by which it reflects on its own thoughts 'and existence, and relation to other 'things, as well as its reasoning and mo-'ral faculties, unfold themselves by de-'grees; so that it is inspired with the va-'rious principles of common sense as with 'the passions of love and resentment, 'when it has occasion for them. Let our author say how this supposition of his could be possible, if ideas of sensation were necessarily included under the head of ideas of reflection, when they are here said to have existed prior to the very power of reflection, or at least to any exercise of that power.

By the way, this hypothesis of the gradual *unfolding* of the powers of the mind very much resembles the gradual *acquisition* of them, from the impressions to which we are exposed. I should have thought that Dr. Reid would hardly have had an idea of real *powers* lying so long dormant as this notion may require some of them to do, while other faculties were awake

awake and vigorous. He will not, I find, assert of *powers* what he does of *ideas*, viz. that they have no existence but when they are in use and exercise.

---

## SECTION V.

*Dr.* Reid's *position, that sensation implies the belief of the present existence of external objects and his view of* Berkley's *theory, particularly considered.*

HAVING replied to our author's capital objections to Mr. Locke's, or the common hypothesis, concerning sensations, ideas and objects, I come to consider what he has farther to advance in support of his own. Now one would imagine *a priori*, that a man who should have assumed the airs and tone that Dr. Reid has given himself through the whole of this treatise, as if he had utterly demolished all the preceding systems of the

the mind, and erected another quite different from any thing that was ever heard or thought of before, would be able to produce ſomething like *poſitive evidence* for it. But, behold, when we have got to the end of theſe *negative arguments*, he has, in fact, nothing more to offer, beſides his own very confident aſſertions (repeated indeed without end, if that would give them any weight) that the thing muſt certainly be as he repreſents it.

Now though I, who do not pretend to advance any hypotheſis of my own, might very reaſonably imitate his example; and, having ſhewn the futility of his objections to the commonly received hypotheſis, content myſelf with leaving things in *ſtatu quo*; yet for the greater ſatisfaction of my readers, I ſhall make a few more obſervations on the ſubject of our author's inſtinctive principles, ſelecting for a more particular examination that by which he ſays *our perceptions neceſſarily imply the belief of the preſent exiſtence of external objects.* There is no one article

of

of his whole ſyſtem of common ſenſe that he can leſs ſcruple to ſubmit to this examination; for there is no one thing that he repeats ſo often, or ſeems to triumph in ſo much, as this; imagining that his method of conſidering the ſubject is an effectual antidote, and the only effectual antidote to all the ſcepticiſm of the preſent age.

Now excepting what our author has ſaid about the abſurdity of Mr. Locke's principles, of which I think I have offered a ſufficient vindication, and of the peculiarly abſurd and dangerous conſequences which he aſcribes to Berkley's theory, and which I ſhall preſently ſhow to be no better founded, all that he ſays amounts to nothing more than this; that he cannot, in his own mind, ſeparate the belief of the exiſtence of external objects from his ſenſations, as thoſe of taſte, touch, ſight, &c. With reſpect to this I would make the following obſervations.

1. There

1. There are many opinions which we know to be acquired, and even founded on prejudice and miſtake, which, however, the fulleſt conviction that they are void of all real foundation cannot eraſe from the mind; the groundleſs *belief*, and *expectation*, founded upon it, being ſo cloſely connected with the idea of certain circumſtances, that no mental power of which we are poſſeſſed can ſeparate them.

Though, for inſtance, Dr. Reid, no doubt, as well as other philoſophers, believes the earth to be ſpherical, and conſequently is ſenſible that no one part of its ſurface can be *uppermoſt* and another part under it; or, that if there were ſuch a thing as an uppermoſt part, every part muſt become ſo in its turn; yet he always conſiders the place on which he ſtands as conſtantly uppermoſt, and conceives of his antipodes as hanging with their heads downwards. Nay he cannot help having an idea of their having a tendency to fall down into the void ſpace below the earth.

He

He may talk as a philoſopher, but I am confident he conceives and thinks as the vulgar do; and though in many things our author appeals to the ſentiments of the vulgar as the teſt of truth, in oppoſition to the philoſophers, I think he will hardly chuſe to do ſo in this caſe. He cannot, however, poſſibly ſeparate in his imagination the idea of a tendency to fall from his idea of the ſituation of the antipodes. Now why may not this be the caſe with reſpect to Berkley's theory, ſo that though we cannot ſeparate the idea of the real exiſtence of external objects and our ſenſations; it may, like the other, be no more than a prejudice, void of all real foundation. As we cannot pretend to diſtinguiſh between our feelings in theſe two caſes, and one of them we know to be fallacious, why may not the other be fallacious alſo? There muſt be ſome *other kind* of evidence beſides *feeling*, to prove that it is not ſo.

Secondly, This ſcheme of Dr. Reid's ſuppoſes that an extraordinary proviſion is made for a *kind* of faith, that is by no means neceſſary for the purpoſe of it, viz. with reſpect to the conduct of life. For a very high degree of probability, not to be diſtinguiſhed in feeling from abſolute certainty, is attainable without it. Now ſince it cannot be denied but that the divine being leaves us to be governed by a kind of faith far inferior to mathematical certainty in things of infinitely more conſequence (in this, however, I do not appeal to Dr. Oſwald) it is abſolutely incredible that he ſhould have implanted in us a peculiar inſtinctive principle, merely for the ſake of giving us a *plenary conviction* with reſpect to this buſineſs, which is comparatively of very trifling conſequence.

Thirdly, Our author's ſcheme has this farther untoward circumſtance attending it, that it ſuppoſes the divine being to have formed us in ſuch a manner, as that we muſt neceſſarily believe what, by our author's own confeſſion, *might not have been true*. For ' no man,' ſays he, p. 85, ' can

'can ſhow by any good argument, that 'all our ſenſations might not have been 'as they are, though no body or quality 'of body had ever exiſted.' Now this I ſhould think to be, upon the face of it, ſo very unlikely to be true, that no perſon who conſiders the caſe can admit of it. For this is very different from thoſe deceptions which neceſſarily ariſe from general laws, and to which all mankind are ſubject; but with reſpect to which it is in their power, by the proper uſe of their faculties, to relieve themſelves.

It appears, therefore, that confident as our author is of the truth and importance of his ſyſtem, he acknowledges it to be founded not on *abſolute* but *relative truth*, ariſing from his conſtitution, which (contrary to what is advanced by his followers Dr. Beattie and Dr. Oſwald) is eſſentially different from that kind of evidence by which we are ſatisfied that two and two are four, which is independent of any *arbitrary conſtitution* whatever.

I wonder

I wonder it ſhould not have a little ſtaggered Dr. Reid, to conſider that his whole ſyſtem muſt fall at once before the fainteſt ſuſpicion, that God may think proper that mankind ſhould be ſubject to deceptions for their good, at which my mind does not ſhudder, when I ſee it to be the neceſſary conſequence of the moſt excellent general laws. Do we not ſee that the bulk of mankind live and die in the belief that the ſun moves round the earth, and of other things in which they are deceived by the teſtimony of their ſenſes? Now let Dr. Reid aſſign a *good reaſon*, why the ſame being who permits his creatures to believe that the ſun moves round the earth, might not permit them to believe that there was a ſun, though, in reality, there ſhould be no ſuch thing; at the ſame time that, by his own immediate power, without the aid of any real ſun, he ſhould afford them all the benefit of light and heat which they had falſely aſcribed to that luminary. I allow it to be as *improbable* as any perſon pleaſes, but the ſuppoſition is certainly not

directly

directly abſurd and *impoſſible*, and this is the only thing in debate.

Fourthly, I wonder that our author ſhould not have attempted ſome ſolution of the phenomena of *dreams*, *reveries*, and *viſions* upon his hypotheſis. In all theſe circumſtances it cannot be denied that men imagine themſelves to be ſurrounded with objects which have no real exiſtence, and yet their ſenſations are not to be diſtinguiſhed from thoſe of men awake; ſo that if *ſenſations, as ſuch*, neceſſarily draw after them the belief of the preſent exiſtence of objects, this belief takes place in dreams, reveries, and viſions, as indeed is the caſe; and if there be a fallacy in theſe caſes, it is certainly *within the compaſs of poſſibility*, that there may be a fallacy in the other alſo.

Notwithſtanding theſe obvious difficulties with which our author's ſcheme is clogged, and which a genius of any order leſs than *the moſt daring* would think to be inſuperable, nothing can exceed the confidence with which he expresses his full persuasion of the truth of it, from the supposed impossibility of believing the contrary, or the supercilious and cavalier manner in which he treats all objections to it.

'I am aware,' says he, p. 291, 'that 'this belief which I have in perception 'stands exposed to the strongest batteries 'of scepticism. But they make no great 'impression upon it. The sceptic asks 'me, why do you believe the existence 'of the external object which you per-'ceive? This belief, Sir, is none of my 'manufacture; it came from the mint of 'nature; it bears her image and super-'scription; and if it is not right, the fault 'is not mine. I even took it upon trust, 'and without suspicion. Reason, says 'the sceptic, is the only judge of truth, 'and you ought to throw off every opi-'nion, and every belief, that is not 'grounded on reason. Well, Sir, why 'should I believe the faculty of reason 'more than that of perception? They 'both

'both came out of the ſame ſhop, and 'were made by the ſame artiſt; and if he 'puts one piece of falſe ware into my 'hands, what ſhould hinder him from 'putting another?'

'Perhaps the ſceptic will agree to diſ-'truſt reaſon, rather than give any credit to 'perception. For, ſays he, ſince by your 'own confeſſion, the object which you 'perceive, and that act of your mind by 'which you perceive it are quite different 'things, the one may exiſt without the 'other; and as the object may exiſt with-'out being perceived, ſo the perception 'may exiſt without an object. There is 'nothing ſo ſhameful in a philoſopher as 'to be deceived, and deluded, and there-'fore you ought firmly to withhold your 'aſſent, and throw off this belief of ex-'ternal objects, which may be all delu-'ſion. For my part, I will never attempt 'to throw it off, and although the ſober 'part of mankind will not be very anxious 'to know any reaſons, yet if they can be 'of uſe to any ſceptic, they are theſe.'

Now, as I do not pretend to rank myſelf with thoſe whom Dr. Reid will call the *ſober part of mankind*, I frankly acknowledge that I have had a little curioſity to look at theſe reaſons.

The firſt I find is, that it is not in his power to believe otherwiſe, which I preſume I have conſidered ſufficiently above.

His ſecond argument is derived from the dangerous conſequences which he aſcribes to Berkley's hypotheſis, and which he expreſſes in that ludicrous and contemptuous manner in which the greateſt part of this *philoſophical treatiſe* is written.

'I think,' ſays he, p. 291, 'it would 'not be prudent to throw off this belief, 'if it were in my power. If nature in- 'tended to deceive me, and impoſe upon 'me by falſe appearances, and I, by my 'great cunning and profound logic, have 'diſcovered the impoſture, prudence 'would

'would dictate to me in this caſe even to 'put up this indignity done me, as qui- 'etly as I could, and not to call her an 'impoſtor to her face, leſt ſhe ſhould be 'even with me in another way. For 'what do I gain by reſenting this injury? 'You ought, at leaſt, not to believe what 'ſhe ſays. This, indeed, ſeems reaſon- 'able, if ſhe intends to impoſe upon me. 'But what is the conſequence. I reſolve 'not to believe my ſenſes. I break my 'noſe againſt a poſt that comes in my 'way; I ſtep into a dirty kennel; and 'after twenty ſuch wiſe and rational ac- 'tions, I am taken up, and clapt into a 'mad-houſe. Now I confeſs I had rather 'make one of the credulous fools whom 'nature impoſes upon, than of thoſe wiſe 'and rational philoſophers, who reſolve 'to withhold aſſent at all this expence.'

But all this profuſion of genuine wit and humour turns upon a groſs miſrepreſentation of Berkley's theory; and it is really a pity that what is ſo excellent in its kind ſhould be thrown away, by being miſplaced.

This misrepresentation and abuse is exactly the conduct of many divines, who charge one another with actually maintaining the supposed consequences of their respective opinions. But this is no *fair* consequence. Berkley did not exclude from his system *sensations* and *ideas*, together with matter, the *necessary connections* that subsist among them, or our *power* over them. He only ascribed them to a *different origin*; so that all the rules of conduct depending upon them are the same on his scheme as on ours. Our philosophical language only is different.

I say there is a post in my way, and I must turn aside, lest I hurt myself by running against it. He, in the same situation, is as apprehensive of danger as myself, though he says he has only the idea of a post before him; for if he do not introduce the idea of avoiding it, he is sensible that he shall experience a very painful sensation, which may bring on other sensations, till death itself ensue. I may smile at his language, but he is consistent

consistent with himself, and his fears have as much foundation as mine.

This representation of Berkley's theory, which is common to Dr. Reid, Dr. Beattie, and Dr. Oswald, and with which they often make themselves and their readers foolishly merry, is exceedingly unjust; but when considered by philosophers, the laugh must rebound upon themselves.

The third reason, as our author is pleased to call it, why he believes in the existence of a material world, or the evidence of his senses, is that he does not find that he has been imposed upon by this belief. 'I find,' says he, p. 293 'that 'without it I must have perished by a 'thousand accidents. I find that without 'it I should have been no wiser now than 'when I was born' &c. &c. &c. But all this goes upon the same misrepresentation with the former argument, and is not, in fact, at all different from it. Besides, a reasonable degree of evidence, which may be attained without this extraordinary, inſtinctive, abſolute, and as our author calls it, *inſpired belief*, is juſt as uſeful for any real purpoſe.

---

## SECTION VI.

### *Mr.* Locke's *doctrine not ſo favourable to* Berkley's *theory as Dr.* Reid's.

IT is by an evident abuſe and perverſion of Mr. Locke's doctrine that Dr. Reid pretends that it is favourable to Biſhop Berkley's notion of there being no material world; when, in reality, our author's own principles are much more favourable to that notion than Mr. Locke's.

'If,' ſays he, p. 42, 'impreſſions and 'ideas are the only objects of thought, 'then heaven and earth, and body and 'ſpirit, and every thing you pleaſe, muſt 'ſignify only impreſſions and ideas, or 'they muſt be words without any meaning.'

But

But it was never ſuppoſed by Mr. Locke, or any other advocate for ideas, that they were more than the *immediate* object of our thoughts, the things of which we are properly ſpeaking *conſcious*, or that we know in the *firſt inſtance*. From them, however, we think we can *infer* the real exiſtence of other things, from which thoſe ideas are derived; and then we can reaſon about thoſe *objects*, as well as about the *ideas* themſelves. In fact, ideas being only the ſigns of external things, we reaſon about the external things themſelves, without ever attending to the ideas which repreſent them, and even without knowing that there are any ſuch things in the mind, till we come to reflect upon the ſubject. In like manner, a perſon may ſee perfectly without ever thinking of his eyes, or indeed knowing that he has any ſuch organs.

Mr. Locke would not, indeed pretend to ſuch an abſolute *demonſtration* of the reality of an external world as Dr. Reid pleads for; but neither is that ſtrict de-

monſtration

monſtration neceſſary. It is quite ſufficient if the ſuppoſition be the eaſieſt hypotheſis for explaining the origin of our ideas. The evidence of it is ſuch that we allow it to be barely poſſible to doubt of it; but that it is as certain as that two and two make four, we do not pretend.

Strongly attached as our author is to this material world of ours, let us ſee whether his own ſyſtem, in other reſpects, be ſufficiently adapted to it. Now it appears to me that his notions of mind, ideas, and external objects, are ſuch as are hardly compatible with one another, that he puts an impaſſable gulph between them, ſo as intirely to prevent their connection or correſpondence; which is all that the biſhop could wiſh in favour of his doctrine.

I take it for granted,' ſays Dr. Reid, p. 381, 'upon the teſtimony of common 'ſenſe, that my mind is a ſubſtance, that 'is, a permanent ſubject of thought, and 'my 'my reaſon convinces me that it is an un-'extended and indiviſible ſubſtance; and 'hence I infer that there cannot be in it any 'thing that reſembles extenſion.' But with equal appearance of truth he might infer that the mind cannot be *affected* by any thing that has extenſion; for how can any thing act upon another but by means of ſome common property? Though, therefore, the divine being has thought proper to create an external world, it can be of no proper uſe to give us ſenſations or ideas. It muſt be he himſelf that impreſſes our minds with the notices of external things, without any *real inſtrumentality* of their own; ſo that the external world is quite a ſuperfluity in the creation. If, therefore, the author of all things be a *wiſe* being, and have made nothing in vain, we may conclude that this external world, which has been the ſubject of ſo much controverſy, can have no exiſtence.

If then we wiſh to preſerve this external world, which is very convenient for many purpoſes, we muſt take care to entertain notions

notions of mind and ideas more compatible with it than thoſe of Dr. Reid.

Our author's fallacious argument from the want of reſemblance between our ideas and external objects leads him into many difficulties. It makes him, in ſeveral reſpects, allow too much to Dr. Berkley, and to come nearer to him than he is aware. And in ſpite of his averſion to the union, and of every thing that he can do or ſay, their common principles will bring them together. 'Our ſenſa-'tions' he ſays, p. 305, 'have no reſem-'blance to external objects, nor can we 'diſcover by our reaſon any neceſſary 'connection between the exiſtence of the 'former and that of the latter. No man,' ſays he, p. 85, 'can ſhew by any good 'argument, that all our ſenſations might 'not have been as they are, though no 'body or quality of body had ever ex-'iſted.' He even ſays, p. 304, 'that 'when we conſider the different attributes 'of *mind* and *body*, they ſeem to be ſo 'different, and ſo unlike, that we can find

'no

'no handle by which one may lay hold
'of the other.'

According to our author, therefore, Berkley's theory is at leaſt *poſſible*; and if, as he ſays, p. 117, 'ſenſations and 'ideas in our minds can reſemble nothing 'but ſenſations and ideas in other minds,' it may well appear *probable*, that they are transferred (as Malebranche, I think, ſuppoſes) immediately from the divine mind to ours, without any real agency of a material world. If I could admit Dr. Reid's premiſes, I think I could hardly help drawing this concluſion from them; eſpecially as nothing can be pleaded for the exiſtence of this ſame material world, but a mere *unaccountable perſuaſion* that it *does* exiſt. This perſuaſion Dr. Reid ſays ariſes from a branch of his new common ſenſe. But if I cannot diſcover or imagine any *end* or *reaſon* why it ſhould exiſt; common ſenſe, in its old and familiar acceptation, would tell me that it does not exiſt at all.

## SECTION VII.

*A sophism of Mr.* Hume's *in pursuance of* Berkley's *theory adopted by Dr.* Reid.

OUR author, struck with a panic fear of scepticism, has been no less misled, and thrown off his guard, by the dangerous sophisms of Mr. Hume, than by the innocent ones of Bishop Berkley,

'The *new system*,' by which he means that of Descartes and Locke, &c. he says, p. 369, 'admits only of the principles 'of common sense as a first principle, and 'pretends by strict argumentation to de-'duce all the rest from it. That our 'thoughts, our sensations, and every thing 'of which we are conscious has a real ex-'istence is admitted in this system as a 'first principle, but every thing else must 'be made evident by the light of reason. 'That the rational issue of this system is 'scepticism, with regard to every thing 'excepting the existence of our ideas, 'and

'and their neceſſary relations, which ap-'pear upon comparing them, is evident. 'For ideas being the only objects of 'thought, and having no exiſtence but 'when we are conſcious of them, it ne-'ceſſarily follows, that there is no object 'of our thought which can have a conti-'nued and permanent exiſtence. Body 'and ſpirit, cauſe and effect, time and 'ſpace, to which we were wont to aſcribe 'an exiſtence independent of our thought, 'all are turned out of exiſtence by this 'ſhort dilemma. Either theſe things are 'ideas of ſenſation or reflection, or they 'are not. If they are ideas of ſenſation 'or reflection, they can have no ex-'iſtence but when we are conſcious of 'them. If they are not ideas of ſenſation 'or reflection, they are words without any 'meaning.' p. 373.

From this pitiful ſophiſm, advanced by Mr. Hume, and deemed unanſwerable by Dr. Reid, have been derived to us all the inſtinctive principles contained in this curious treatiſe. For being determined

at

at all adventures to maintain the reality of body and ſpirit, cauſe and effect, time and ſpace, &c. and the old theory of the mind not being, in his opinion, ſufficient for the purpoſe, a new one muſt be found; and if nothing elſe can be had, ſtill the good things above mentioned muſt be retained, though we can ſay nothing in their favour but *they are ſo becauſe they are ſo*, which is Dr. Reid's common ſenſe, and his ſhort irrefragable argument.

But if, inſtead of ſuch a *plenary aſſurance* as only this new common ſenſe promiſes, he would have been content with a *reaſonable degree of evidence* for the reality of all the things above mentioned, the old hypotheſis would have been quite ſufficient. It ſuits every caſe of ſenſations and ideas; and therefore, according to the received rules of philoſophizing, has a juſt claim to be admitted.

That *mind* exiſts I have the very ſame reaſon to believe as I have that *body* exiſts; ſince it is only by that name that I diſtinguiſh

diſtinguiſh that to which certain powers and properties, of which I am conſcious, as *perception*, *memory*, *will*, &c. belong.

I am ſurprized that it ſhould have been ſo readily admitted, that even ideas have no exiſtence but when we are conſcious of them. We have juſt the ſame reaſon to believe the identity of an idea, as that of a tree, that of any external body, or that of our own minds themſelves. The idea that I have of my wife or child to-day as much reſembles the idea I had of them yeſterday, though ſome hours of ſound ſleep have intervened, as my houſe of to-day reſembles my houſe of yeſterday. In this caſe I only judge by the reſemblance of my ideas of it; and if the ideas of my houſe yeſterday and to-day were not the ſame, I ſhould have no medium by which to prove the identity of the houſe.

## SECTION VIII.

*Cafes of the affociation of ideas which had efcaped the attention of Dr.* Reid.

I Have obferved that one of the fallacious mediums of proof which our author makes much ufe of, in order to prove that we judge and act from original inftinct, and not by any acquired power, is our ignorance of the means by which any action is performed, and our having made thofe judgments, and performed thofe actions, prior to experience. In the former of thefe cafes he draws *wrong conclufions* from his premifes, and in the latter I have no doubt but he is miftaken with refpect to the *facts* from which he argues. I fhall now prefent my readers with fome inftances of both thefe kinds of fallacy.

‘ In fome of the voluntary, as well as ‘ the involuntary motions’ (which Dr. Reid exemplifies by that of the parallel motion of of both the eyes, which he ſays takes place previous to cuſtom, in conſequence of ſome natural inſtinct) 'many muſcles,' he ſays, p. 187, 'which have no material tie or 'connection, act in concert, each of them 'being taught to play its part in exact 'time and meaſure; yet we ſee ſuch ac'tions no leſs ſkilfully and regularly per'formed in children, and thoſe who know 'not that they have ſuch muſcles, than 'in the moſt ſkilful anatomiſt and phyſio'logiſt.'

From theſe premiſes he might juſt as well have inferred, that we have no ſuch muſcles. In fact, our *knowledge* of the particular muſcles employed in any motion is of no conſequence whatever to the *performance* of it. Nature has ſufficiently provided for that in the ſimple power of aſſociation, whereby one idea or motion introduces another aſſociated idea or motion mechanically, and without the exertion of any voluntary power in us: and this is equally the caſe whether volition was employed in forming the original aſſociation, or not.

It was my misfortune to have the idea of darkneſs, and the ideas of inviſible malignant ſpirits and apparitions very cloſely connected in my infancy; and to this day, notwithſtanding I believe nothing of thoſe inviſible powers, and conſequently of their connection with darkneſs, or any thing elſe, I cannot be perfectly eaſy in every kind of ſituation in the dark, though I am ſenſible I gain ground upon this prejudice continually.

I likewiſe ſometimes amuſe myſelf with playing on a flute, which I did not learn very early, ſo that I have a perfect remembrance that I exerted an expreſs voluntary power every time that I covered any particular hole with my finger. But though I am no great proficient on the inſtrument, there are ſome tunes which I now very often play without ever attending to my fingers, or explicitly to the tune. I have even played in concert, and, as I was informed, perfectly in tune, when I have been ſo abſent, that, excepting at the beginning, I did not recollect that I had been playing at all. The ſame is alſo

frequently

frequently the caſe with perſons who are reading.

Now, reaſoning as Dr. Reid does, I ſhould conclude that, in this caſe, no ſkill, acquired by habit, was employed, but that my fingers were guided by ſome original inſtinctive principle; and if I had been able to do this earlier than my remembrance of any thing, I muſt have ſaid that this was one of thoſe powers, which, being latent in the mind, was called forth by proper circumſtances. Whereas, I think it more natural to ſay, that the aſſociation between the ideas of certain ſounds and the cauſe of certain motions of the fingers became in time ſo perfect, that the one introduced the other, without any attention; the intervening expreſs volition, previous to each motion, having been gradually excluded. Facts of this kind demonſtrate that the power of aſſociation is ſo great, and ſo extenſive, that even whole trains and very long trains of ideas, are by this means ſo connected, that if the firſt take place, all the reſt will follow of courſe, without our giving any attention to them, and even while we are attending to other things, and things of a very different nature.

'Who' ſays our author, p. 188, 'taught 'all the muſcles that are concerned in 'ſucking, in ſwallowing our food, in 'breathing, and in ſeveral natural expul-'ſions, to act their part in ſuch regular 'order, and exact meaſure? It was not 'cuſtom ſurely.' But in theſe, and many ſuch inſtances, it is exceedingly probable that the actions of the muſcles were originally *automatic*, having been ſo placed by our maker, that at firſt they are ſtimulated and contract mechanically whenever their action is requiſite; and though the muſcles themſelves have no connection, their nerves are connected, and they may be ſo ſituated, that the ſame cauſes of contraction ſhall neceſſarily affect ſeveral of them at the ſame time, or in a certain regular ſucceſſion. In ſome of the actions to which Dr. Reid refers, we ſee evident marks of ſuch a mechanical progreſs;

greſs; and more knowledge of nature and phyſiology may lead to the diſcovery of more of them; provided this ſyſtem of having recourſe at once to *ultimate cauſes* does not prevent men from giving proper attention to them.

The fæces are at firſt expelled involuntarily, and a voluntary power over the muſcles which are ſubſervient to that operation is evidently acquired gradually. The ſame is the progreſs in the action of blowing the noſe. Children have not, naturally, the leaſt notion how to do it, any more than they have how to walk. The action of *ſucking*, I am alſo confident, from my own obſervations, is not natural but acquired; and ſo I believe are all the actions which Dr. Reid and others, who judge ſuperficially in theſe caſes, refer to inſtinct; and with reſpect to which I would refer him to Dr. Hartley, who has written expreſsly, and pretty largely upon theſe ſubjects.

With reſpect to ſeeing objects erect by means of inverted images, Dr. Reid ſays,

p. 151, that 'the premifes from which
' all mankind are fuppofed to draw the
' conclufion (referring to the Cartefian
' hypothefis) never entered into the minds
' of the far greater part, but are abfolutely
' unknown to them. In order to fee ob-
' jects erect, according to the principles
' of Kepler, we muft previoufly know
' that the rays of light come from the
' object in ftraight lines, we muft know
' that the rays from the different points
' of the object crofs one another before
' they form pictures upon the retina, and
' laftly we muft know that thefe pictures
' are really inverted. Now though all
' thefe things be true, and known to phi-
' lofophers, yet they are abfolutely un-
' known to the far greateft part of man-
' kind; nor is it poffible that they who
' are abfolutely ignorant of them fhould
' reafon from them, and build conclufions
' upon them.'

I do not know how this may affect others, but it really furprizes me to hear a man of any underftanding reafon fo very weakly.

weakly. To *feel* a thing, to be *affected* by it, and to be influenced and directed in our future conduct by that feeling, certainly cannot require that we should *know* the connection there is between the objects and our perceptions of them; but simply that there *be* that connection. They who are the most ignorant of the laws of vision are nevertheless *subject* to them; so that their retinas, optic nerves, brains, and minds, are differently affected in consequence of the rays of light coming in straight lines, crossing one another before they reach the retina; and pictures are actually formed there, whether we know of them or not. All men, even the most ignorant, find by experience which way they must turn their heads and eyes to look for any object by which they are impressed; and these associations are so frequent, that we pass immediately and mechanically, from the one to the other; so that the moment we perceive an object we throw our heads and direct our eyes into the most proper position for the distinct view of it. If,

for

ſor this purpoſe, we find that we muſt turn our heads and eyes upwards, we ſay the object is above us; but if we muſt turn them downwards, we ſay it is below us, without knowing any thing farther about the matter.

---

## SECTION IX.

*Conceſſions of Dr.* Reid, *and other circumſtances, which might have led him to have recourſe to the* aſſociation of ideas, *rather than to his* inſtinctive principles.

THOUGH it is apparent, from the whole of Dr. Reid's treatiſe, that he has given very little attention to the doctrine of the *aſſociation of ideas* (far leſs than its obvious importance demanded) yet, in ſome caſes, it could not poſſibly eſcape his notice; and he has expreſſed himſelf in ſuch a manner with reſpect to ſome of them, as makes me wonder that he did not ſee that more uſe might be made

made of it, and that the phenomena would admit of a very easy explanation, without having recourse to his instinctive principles; which ought to have been kept for great emergencies only, *nodi deo vindice digni*.

I am particularly surprized that Dr. Reid should hesitate to acknowledge that our judgment of the unity of an object seen with both eyes is acquired, when he owns that we do acquire a judgment which appears to me to be exactly similar to it.

He says, p. 363, that 'Dr. Smith justly 'attributes to custom that well known 'fallacy in vision, whereby a button 'pressed with two opposite sides of two 'contiguous fingers, laid across, is felt 'double.' He adds, that, 'as custom 'produces this phenomenon, so a con-'trary custom destroys it. For if a man 'frequently accustoms himself to feel the 'button with his fingers across, it will at 'last be felt single, as I have found by experience.'

'experience.' Now why may not cuſtom do the ſame thing with reſpect to viſion? It is evident, from theſe ſimilar facts, that it is within the *power* of cuſtom, and of the aſſociation of ideas to do it. I can ſee no more occaſion for *naturally correſponding points* of the retina, than for naturally correſponding places in the fingers.

But he ſays, p. 261, 'If ſingle viſion 'is the effect of cuſtom, it muſt appear 'very ſtrange that not one inſtance has 'been found of a perſon who had acquired 'the habit of ſeeing objects ſingle with 'both eyes, while they were directed in 'any other manner,' viz. than ſo that the centers correſpond. But are not all our eyes ſimilar, and are they not all expoſed to ſimilar influences; and what can reſult from this but uniformity in our rules of judging by their affections?

Our author allows, p. 188, that 'although it appears to be by natural inſtinct that both eyes are always turned the

'the ſame way, there is ſtill ſome latitude 'left for cuſtom. Nature has wiſely left 'us the power of varying the paralleliſm 'of the eyes a little, ſo that we can di-'rect them to the ſame point, whether 'remote or near. This no doubt is 'learned by cuſtom, and accordingly we 'ſee that it is a long time before children 'get this habit in perfection.' But according to Dr. Reid's general rule, we ought to have referred this caſe alſo to original inſtinct, becauſe we are poſſeſſed of this power prior to any experience that we can remember, and we are not conſcious of the means by which we exert it, or indeed know that we do any ſuch thing at all. Previous to reflection, we imagine that we have ſimply a power of ſeeing diſtinctly at different diſtances. We are conſcious of nothing farther, and therefore, according to this new mode of philoſophizing, we may reaſonably acquieſce in the fact, and call the power original and inſtinctive; in other words, one of the many branches of the new common ſenſe.

'Though

'Though we are not conſcious,' ſays Dr. Reid, p. 310, 'of the motions we "perform in order to fit the eyes to the 'diſtance of objects, we are conſcious of 'the effort employed in producing theſe 'motions, and probably have ſome ſenſa-'tion which accompanies them, to which "we give as little attention as to other 'ſenſations.' But unleſs the diſtance be conſiderable, we are not conſcious of uſing any effort at all. Beſides, according to this new mode of reaſoning, how can the mind employ the muſcles that are requiſite to make this effort, when it has no knowledge of them, or indeed of the nature and mode of action of any muſcle whatever?

As our author generally refers that to inſtinct which has been acquired by experience and the aſſociation of ideas, ſo he gives to cuſtom and experience what properly belongs to reaſoning and judgment; though here alſo his own conceſſions might have led him to a right judgment in the ſeveral caſes.

'When

'When I hear a certain ſound,' he ſays, p. 71. 'I conclude immediately without 'reaſoning, that a coach paſſes by. There 'are no premiſes by which this concluſion is inferred by any rules of logic. 'It is the effect of a principle of our nature common to us with the brutes.' This principle he before called cuſtom or experience.

In what different lights may the ſame thing be ſeen by different perſons, according as their different hypotheſes incline them to regard it. In this very mental operation, or proceſs, in which Dr. Reid can find no trace of reaſoning or judgment, I think I ſee every part of a complete argument; and even that facility, and readineſs in paſſing from the premiſes to the concluſion, which argues the very perfection of intellect in the caſe. For in my idea it is only in conſequence of the mode of reaſoning being very familiar, that the mind jumps with ſuch rapidity to the final judgment, that it requires ſome attention to diſcover the medium of proof.

The

The proceſs, when properly unfolded, is as follows: The ſound I now hear is, in all reſpects, ſuch as I have formerly heard, which appeared to be occaſioned by a coach paſſing by, *ergo*, this is alſo occaſioned by a coach. Into this ſyllogiſm it appears to me that the mental proceſs that Dr. Reid mentions may fairly be reſolved; and I am ſurpriſed he ſhould not have thought ſo himſelf, when he expreſsly allows, p. 128, that 'the operations of the 'mind may be ſo ſubtle, that we draw 'concluſions without ever perceiving that 'the premiſes entered the mind.' This conceſſion, which is a very juſt and reaſonable one, certainly overturns the very foundation of his argument in the preceding caſe.

In this one caſe Dr. Oſwald, more conſiſtently with the ſyſtem, decides againſt his maſter. 'The ſuppoſition,' ſays he, vol. 2, p. 56, 'of a proceſs of reaſoning which paſſes ſo quickly through 'the mind as not to be perceived, is al'together arbitrary; and arbitrary ſup'poſitions are extremely injurious to truth,

'and

'and give birth to that multitude of chi-'merical hypotheses by which mankind 'have been misled.'

If a dog can form the same conclusion from the same premises, I would not scruple to say that the dog reasoned as well and as justly as myself. I see no reason to deny brute animals the power of reasoning concerning the objects about which they are conversant. They certainly act as *consequentially*, as if they reasoned.

Again, upon our author's mistaking a seagull for a man on horseback, he says, p. 319, 'the mistake and the correction 'of it are both so sudden, that we are at 'a loss whether to call them by the name 'of judgment, or by that of simple per-'ception.' In fact, these things run insensibly into one another.

Lastly, he acknowledges, p. 154, that 'it must be extremely difficult to distin-'guish the immediate and natural objects 'of sight, from the conclusions which we 'have been accuftomed to draw from 'them.'

---

## SECTION X.

*Of Dr.* Reid's *principle of credulity, and his idea of the principles of induction, and analogy.*

THAT any man fhould imagine that a peculiar inftinctive principle was neceffary to explain our giving credit to the relations of others, appears to me, who have been ufed to fee things in a different light, very extraordinary; and yet this doctrine is advanced by Dr. Reid, and adopted by Dr. Beattie. But really what our author fays in favour of it is hardly deferving of the flighteft notice.

'If credulity,' he fays, p. 340, 'were 'the effect of reafoning and experience, 'it muft grow up and gather ftrength in 'the fame proportion as reafon and ex- 'perience

'perience do. But if it is the gift of 'nature, it will be the ſtrongeſt in child'hood, and limited and reſtrained by ex'perience; and the moſt ſuperficial view 'of human life ſhows that this laſt is re'ally the caſe, and not the firſt.'

This reaſoning is exceedingly fallacious. It is a long time before a child hear any thing but truth, and therefore it can *expect* nothing elſe. The contrary would be abſolutely miraculous. Falſehood is a *new circumſtance*, which he likewiſe comes to expect in proportion as he has been taught by experience to expect it. What evidence can we poſſibly have of any thing being neceſſarily connected with experience and derived from it, beſides its never being prior to it, always conſequent upon it, and exactly in proportion to it?

I ſhall now conſider what our author ſays of the nature of reaſoning by *induction*, and *analogy*. 'If,' ſays he, p. 340, 'a certain degree of cold freezes water 'to-day, and has been known to do ſo in 'all time paſt, we have no doubt but the 'ſame degree of cold will freeze water 'to-morrow, or a year hence. When I 'compare the idea of cold, with that of 'water hardened into a tranſparent ſolid 'body, I can perceive no connection be-'tween them. No man can ſhew the one 'to be the neceſſary effect of the other. 'No man can give a ſhadow of a reaſon 'why nature has conjoined them. But 'do we not learn that conjunction from 'experience? True, experience informs 'us that they have been conjoined in time 'paſt, but no man ever had any expe-'rience of what is future; and this is the 'very queſtion to be reſolved. How 'come we to believe that the future will 'be like the paſt. Children and ideots 'have the belief of the continuance of 'the preſent courſe of nature as ſoon as 'they know that fire will burn them. It 'muſt, therefore, be the effect of inſtinct 'not of reaſon.'

But experience does a great deal more than Dr. Reid here ſuppoſes. It not only informs us that cold and freezing have been conjoined in time paſt, but alſo that what is now time *paſt*, was once *future*; and therefore that there is no more reaſon to ſuſpect that cold will not freeze water now, than there was to doubt yeſterday that it would freeze it to-day. It is only puzzling the queſtion to conſider time as *paſt* or *future* in this caſe. We alſo find by experience that we have not hitherto been deceived in our expectation that the future will be like the paſt in former inſtances, and therefore cannot have any ſuſpicion of being deceived in a ſimilar expectation in other inſtances. It is really aſtoniſhing that any man ſhould aſk the queſtion that Dr. Reid does here, 'How came we to believe that the future will be like the paſt? It is certainly ſufficient to ſay in anſwer to this. Have we not always found it to be ſo? and therefore, how can we ſuſpect the contrary? Though no man has had any experience of what *is* future, every man has had experience of what *was* future. Every ſtep that I take among this writer's ſophiſms raiſes my aſtoniſhment higher than before.

He farther ſays, p. 347, 'If any reader 'ſhould imagine that the inductive prin- 'ciple may be reſolved into what philo- 'ſophers uſually call aſſociation of ideas, 'let him obſerve that by this principle 'natural ſigns are not aſſociated with 'ideas only, but with the belief of the 'things ſignified. Now this can with no 'propriety be called an aſſociation of 'ideas, unleſs ideas and belief be one 'and the ſame thing.'

This appears to me to be a mere quibble, for not only may *ideas*, properly ſo called, but every thing that is *mental*, as *belief*, and every other operation or affection of the mind, and even the immediate cauſe of muſcular motion, be the ſubject of aſſociation, as we ſee it to be in fact. Not to ſay that *belief*, as Dr. Hartley has explained it, conſiſts of ideas, and

is

is, in fact, nothing but a complex idea, or feeling.

I could have had no conception that a professed enemy to scepticism, as Dr. Reid is, should himself be so sceptical as he is with respect to many of the most uncontroverted maxims of philosophy. But, indeed, it is no uncommon thing to charge another with our own peculiar failings, and to see a mote in our brother's eye, when we cannot discern a beam in our own. And as scepticism and credulity go hand in hand with unbelievers, so they do with Dr. Reid. Where all the rest of the world see the most closely connected chain of reasoning, he is always ready to suspect that some link is wanting, and as ready to supply the imaginary defect, not with another link, but with something that is no proper part of a chain, but some invisible power to keep the two parts together.

He is so eager to find *arbitrary connections* between objects and sensations, and between ſenſations and judgment, that he ſometimes overlooks the moſt neceſſary connections of things. He ſays, p. 163, that ' the material impreſſion upon the ' retina, by means of the rays of light, ' ſuggeſts colour, and the poſition of ſome ' external object; but no man can give a ' reaſon why the ſame material impreſſion ' might not have ſuggeſted ſound, or ſmell, ' or either of theſe, along with the poſi- ' tion of the object. And ſince there is ' no neceſſary connection between theſe ' two things, it might, if it had ſo pleaſed ' our creator, have ſuggeſted one of them ' without the other.' But, it is obvious to remark, that then *rays of light* muſt not have been made uſe of, for theſe *neceſſarily* ſuggeſt both colour and form.

# SECTION XI.

*Of the natural signs of the passions.*

ONE would think that a man must never have heard of the general principle of the *association of ideas*, who could possibly take it into his head that certain features, modulations of the voice, and attitudes of the body, require any other principle, in order to suggest the idea and belief of certain thoughts, purposes, and dispositions of mind. Dr. Reid indeed asserts, in proof of this, that 'an infant 'may be put into a fright by an angry 'countenance, and soothed again by smiles 'and blandishments,' p. 89. Now I have had children of my own, and have made many observations and experiments of this kind upon them, and upon this authority I do not hesitate absolutely to deny the fact with respect to them; and I have no doubt but that the same is the case with respect to all other infants; unless those of Dr. Reid should be as different from mine

mine as are our notions of human nature. But nature, I believe, is pretty uniform in her operations and productions, how differently soever we may conceive of them.

Dr. Reid talks of an *infant*, being put into a fright. On the contrary, I assert that an infant (unless by an infant he should mean a child who has had a good deal of experience, and of course has made many observations on the connections of things) is absolutely incapable of terror. I am positive that no child ever showed the least symptom of fear or apprehension, till he had actually received hurts, and had felt pain; and that children have no fear of any particular person or thing, but in consequence of some connection between that person or thing and the pain they have felt.

If any instinct of this kind was more necessary than another, it would be the *dread of fire*. But every body must have observed that infants show no sign of any such thing; for they will as readily put their

their finger to the flame of a candle as to any thing elſe, till they have been burned. But after ſome painful experience of this kind their dread of fire becomes one of Dr. Reid's original inſtinctive principles, and it is as quick and as effectual in its operations as the very beſt of them.

I, moreover, do not heſitate to ſay, that if it were poſſible always to beat and terrify a child with a placid countenance, ſo as never to aſſume that appearance but in thoſe circumſtances, and always to ſooth him with what we call an angry countenance, this natural and neceſſary connection of ideas that Dr. Reid talks of would be reverſed, and we ſhould ſee the child frighted with a ſmile, and delighted with a frown.

In fact, there is no more reaſon to believe that a child is naturally afraid of a frown, than he is afraid of being in the dark; and of this children certainly diſcover no ſign, till they have either found ſomething diſagreeable to them in the dark,

dark, or have been told that there is ſomething dreadful in it.

---

## SECTION XII.

*Of the judgment we form concerning the ſeat of pain.*

IT alſo appears to me that a man muſt be ſtrangely prepoſſeſſed in favour of inſtinctive principles who ſhould think of having recourſe to them for diſtinguiſhing the parts of our bodies affected with particular pleaſures or pains, when the caſe is ſo eaſily explained by the general laws of aſſociation, aided by experience.

'The ſenſation of pain,' Dr. Reid ſays, p. 209. 'is no doubt in the mind, and can-'not be ſaid to have any relation, from its 'own nature, to any part of the body. 'But this ſenſation by our conſtitution 'gives a perception of ſome particular 'part

'part of our body whoſe diſorder cauſes 'the uneaſy ſenſation. If it were not ſo, 'a man who never before felt either the 'gout or tooth ach, when he is firſt ſeized 'with the gout in his toe might miſtake 'it for the tooth ach.'

Now this, I believe, would be the caſe if a man had never before had any ſenſation of any kind, either in his toe or in his tooth. For though Dr. Reid ſays that judgments of this kind are antecedent to all experience, I am poſitive he can have no authority from fact for the aſſertion, or for believing that an infant can diſtinguiſh the ſeat of any ſenſation, or ſo much as know to which of his organs to refer any of them, the firſt time that they are perceived. Indeed, there is no ſort of *occaſion* for any ſuch early knowledge of this kind; for though the very firſt time that a child ſhould make uſe of his ears or noſe, he ſhould not know which of them it was that was affected by a ſmell or a ſound, he would ſoon acquire that knowledge by experience; finding himſelf re-

lieved

lieved by ſtopping his noſe when he perceived a diſagreeable ſmell, and by ſtopping his ears when he perceived a diſagreeable ſound.

In the ſame manner in which we learn to refer the ſeveral ſenſations to their proper organs, we learn to refer pains and impreſſions of all kinds to the places from which the nerves convey them. If Dr. Reid has ever made obſervations upon children, he muſt have obſerved that they do this in a very imperfect manner, making many miſtakes, and growing more perfect in the exerciſe by degrees.

Even men cannot accurately diſtinguiſh the part of the body affected with pain without the aſſiſtance of ſight, in thoſe parts which have not been the ſeat of any very diſtinguiſhable ſenſation. Let the experiment be made by pricking the part, and requiring the perſon to put the tip of his finger exactly upon it, when he is blindfolded.

Of

Of the ſeat of *internal pains* mankind in general have very little knowledge. But in this reſpect alſo men improve by obſervation and experience, and thoſe who have had the moſt experience have the moſt accurate knowledge of this kind, as is the caſe of all other knowledge acquired by experience. Let Dr. Reid apply to this caſe his own obſervations concerning the ſenſe of credulity.

From the whole of Dr. Reid's reaſoning on theſe ſubjects, one would think that he had never heard of ſuch things as *nerves* proceeding from all the different parts of the body to the brain, all appropriated to their reſpective uſes, ſuch as the optic nerves, the auditory nerves, the olfactory nerves, each of which convey ſenſations of different kinds, entering the brain at different places; but that the buſineſs of ſenſation and perception was performed in ſome ſtrange arbitrary manner without them, or any thing of the kind.

## SECTION XIII.

### *Miscellaneous observations.*

I Shall close these animadversions on Dr. Reid's performance with a few miscellaneous articles which shew either the extreme inattention of our author, in condemning others for faults of which he himself is guilty, claiming discoveries which have really nothing in them, or making great boasts when he appears to have been exceedingly ignorant with respect to the subject of which he writes, and the history of it.

Dr. Reid joins in the general laugh at Descartes's argument to prove his own existence from an act of his mind, viz. *doubting*, p. 11. 'For he takes his ex-'istence for granted in this argument, and 'proves nothing at all.' Yet this author himself argues in a manner exactly similar to this of Descartes. 'No man,' says he, p. 39, 'can conceive or believe smelling 'to 'to exiſt of itſelf without a mind, or 'ſomething that has the power of ſmell- 'ing,' and p. 48, 'It appears to be an 'undeniable fact, that, from thought or 'ſenſation, all mankind, conſtantly and 'invariably, from the firſt dawning of re- 'flection, do infer a power or faculty of 'thinking, and a permanent being, or 'mind, to which that faculty belongs.' Though, how this is conſiſtent with what he had ſaid juſt before, viz. that 'the 'belief of our exiſtence precedes all rea- 'ſoning and experience,' I do not ſee.

Certainly the firſt thing that the mind attends to is not *itſelf*, but the things that affect it, or operate upon it. We firſt perceive ſome *property* of every thing before we think of the thing itſelf. Let Dr. Reid, or any other perſon, ſay how the exiſtence of the mind muſt be evidenced but by its affections or operations. Our author even allows that a perſon may have exiſted a conſiderable time without any power of reflection, and conſequently without having an idea of his own ex-

 iſtence.

iſtence. In reality we ſmile at Deſcartes's argument, not becauſe it is an inconcluſive or improper one, but becauſe the thing to be proved is ſo evident, that it needs no proof.

Our author argues largely, p. 135, in favour of the opinion of the vulgar, that colour is a quality of bodies. Of this he makes a great parade, as of ſome very ſerious buſineſs; but I ſhall not argue the matter ſeriouſly with him, becauſe I take it for granted he has ſeen optical experiments, and therefore cannot poſſibly differ from me except in words. I ſhall only obſerve with reſpect to the ſubject, that the vulgar are eaſily brought to acknowledge their miſtake, and never fail to expreſs their ſurprize, as at a real diſcovery, and what was utterly inconſiſtent with their former notions of the matter, when they are ſhewn pieces of white paper aſſuming all the colours of the rainbow by means of a priſm, without any real change in the paper. This has convinced every perſon to whom I have ever ſhewed

ſhewed the experiment that colour is in the *rays of light*, and not in the body.

'Nothing,' ſays our author, p. 167, 'ſhews more clearly our indiſpoſition to 'attend to viſible figure, and viſible ex-'tenſion, than this, that, although ma-'thematical reaſoning is no leſs applicable 'to them than to tangible figure and 'extenſion; yet they have intirely eſcaped 'the notice of mathematicians.

By viſible figure, &c. our author means the projection of the forms of external objects on the concave bottom of the eye. But to what *purpoſe* would it have been to have taken any pains with the ſubject, when it can be of no poſſible *uſe*, and all that we have really any thing to do with are the properties of the *things* of which theſe images are merely the *ſigns*. No man who had any thing ſeri-ous to attend to would ever think of it. I do not remember ever to have ſeen a more egregious piece of ſolemn trifling than the chapter which our author calls *the geometry of visibles* and his account of the *Idomenians*, as he terms those imaginary beings who had no ideas of substance but from sight. Besides, our author acknowledges that the figures upon the retina differ exceedingly little from the real figures which they represent.

Another affectation of originality we see in what our author says concerning the idea of *hardness*. 'The sensation of hardness,' he says, p. 83, 'is so much unknown, as never to have been the object of thought and reflection, nor to have been honoured with a name in any language. May we not hence conclude that the knowledge of the human faculties is but in its infancy?'

Now I see nothing particularly *hard*, to use a pun, in the case of this same idea of hardness. Indeed, it is very rarely that we bestow a name upon the *idea* of any thing. It is very well if the thing itself have got a name; for many are obliged to go without names. But though I shall not

not take the trouble to look into Mr. Locke for the purpose, I make no doubt but that he, and many others, have mentioned the idea of hardness among other abstract ideas, of much more importance, without confounding it with the hard substance that occasioned the idea. At least Dr. Reid's observation does not strike me as any thing either new, or at all important.

That our author is extremely ignorant of what has been written by others on the subject of the human mind, is evident, not only from his total silence concerning Dr. Hartley (whose name, however, appears to have reached Scotland; for his work is quoted with some degree of respect by Dr. Beattie) but from his gross mistake concerning the hints that Newton and others have dropped on the subject.

'About the time of Dr. Briggs,' he says, p. 278, 'the system of the nerves 'was thought to be a stringed instrument, 'composed of vibrating chords, each of 'which had its proper tenſion and tone.' I ſhall not explain to our author what kind of vibration was ſuppoſed to affect the nerves, that I may give him an opportunity of getting a little more knowledge of his ſubject by looking into Newton or Hartley himſelf. But this I will venture to ſay, that ſuch groſs ignorance in a profeſſor of this very ſubject, in ſo conſiderable an univerſity, which has hitherto been diſtinguiſhed for the real eminence of its profeſſors in that department, is diſgraceful to himſelf and to the univerſity. I will even venture to call upon Dr. Reid to name any writer (that has ever had the leaſt ſhadow of reputation) who ſeriouſly maintained that the ſyſtem of the nerves does reſemble *a ſtringed inſtrument, compoſed of vibrating chords.* If any ſuch hypotheſis was ever advanced, I own, it has eſcaped my notice.

To treat with contempt, as Dr. Reid does, every hypotheſis that has been propoſed, and to offer another ſtill more abſurd, merely to laugh at it, and to turn the whole

whole ſubject into ridicule, certainly does not become a philoſopher, who means to promote an inquiry into the powers of nature. I can compare Dr. Reid's conduct in this caſe to nothing but that of the dog in the manger; for he manifeſtly has no knowledge of the ſubject himſelf, and does every thing in his power to prevent others from knowing any thing about it, or inquiring into it.

To give my reader an idea of our author's talent for irony, and at the ſame time to afford him a little reſpite from metaphyſical reaſoning, I ſhall ſubjoin his account of this new hypotheſis of the uſe of the nerves. After enumerating and laughing at every other hypotheſis, he ſays, p. 278,

'These, I think, are all the engines 'into which the nervous ſyſtem has been 'moulded by philoſophers, for conveying 'the images of ſenſible things from the 'organ to the ſenſorium. And for all 'that we know of the matter every man 'may freely chuſe what he thinks fitteſt 'for the purpoſe; for from fact and ex-'periment no one of them can claim pre-'ference to another. Indeed, they all 'ſeem ſo unhandy engines for carrying 'images, that a man would be tempted 'to invent a new one.

'Since then a blind man may gueſs as 'well in the dark as one that ſees, I beg 'leave to offer another conjecture touch-'ing the nervous ſyſtem, which I hope 'will anſwer the purpoſe as well as thoſe 'we have mentioned, and which recom-'mends itſelf by its ſimplicity. Why 'may not the optic nerves, for inſtance, 'be made up of empty tubes, opening 'their mouths wide enough to receive the 'rays of light which form the image up-'on the retina, and gently conveying 'them ſafe, and in their proper order, to 'the very ſeat of the ſoul, until *they flaſh* '*in her face**? It is eaſy for an ingeni-'ous philoſopher to fit the caliber of thoſe 'empty tubes to the diameter of the par-

* A very expreſſive and elegant phraſe.

'ticles of light, ſo as they ſhall receive 'no groſſer kind of matter. And if theſe 'rays ſhould be in danger of miſtaking 'their way, an expedient may alſo be 'found to prevent this. For it requires 'no more than to beſtow upon the tubes 'of the nervous ſyſtem a periſtaltic mo- 'tion, like that of the alimentary tube.

'It is a peculiar advantage of this hy- 'potheſis, that, although all philoſophers 'believe that the ſpecies or images of 'things are conveyed by the nerves to 'the ſoul, yet none of their hypotheſes ſhew 'how this may be done. For how can 'the images of ſound, taſte, ſmell, co- 'lour, figure, and all ſenſible qualities, 'be made out of the vibrations of muſi- 'cal chords, or the undulation of animal 'ſpirits, or of æther? We ought not to 'ſuppoſe means inadequate to the end. 'Is it not as philoſophical, and more in- 'telligible, to conceive, that as the ſto- 'mach receives its food, ſo the ſoul re- 'ceives her images by a kind of nervous 'deglutition? I might add, that we need only

'only continue this periſtaltic motion of 'the nervous tubes from the ſenſorium to 'the extremities of the nerves that ſerve 'the muſcles, in order to account for muſ-'cular motion.

'Thus nature will be conſonant to her-'ſelf, and as ſenſation will be the convey-'ance of the ideal aliment to the mind, ſo 'muſcular motion will be the expulſion 'of the recrementitious part of it. For 'who can deny that the images of things 'conveyed by ſenſation may, after due 'concoction, become fit to be thrown off 'by muſcular motion? I only give hints 'of theſe things to the ingenious, hoping 'that in time this hypotheſis may be 'wrought up into a ſyſtem, as truly philo-'ſophical as that of animal ſpirits, or the 'vibration of nervous fibres. To be 'ſerious'————

To be ſerious then. By ſome perſons all this may be thought very ingenious and clever, the irony delicate, and the expreſſion elegant. But while ſome laugh

*with*

*with* the writer, others may be more diſpoſed to laugh *at* him, both for his ignorance and his buffoonery. I ſhall only ſay that if I have the leaſt notion of what the true *ſpirit of philoſophy* is, this is the very reverſe of it; and that ſuch a mode of writing ought to be treated with indignation and contempt.

Our author's *concluſion*, as well as his *dedication*, which, though printed firſt, ſuppoſes the book to have been written before it, ſhews a perſuaſion of his having done great things, though his ſtyle is unlike that of Horace or Ovid, *Jamque Opus exegi*——He imagined, I ſuppoſe, that he had thrown many *new* lights upon the ſubject of human nature, by throwing down the *old* ones erected by Deſcartes and Locke.

'I intended to have examined more 'particularly and fully this doctrine of 'the exiſtence of ideas, or images of things 'in the mind, and likewiſe another doc- 'trine which is founded upon it, to wit, 'that

'that judgment or belief is nothing but a 'perception of the agreement or disagree-'ment of our ideas, but having already 'shewn that the operations of the mind 'which we have examined give no coun-'tenance to either of these doctrines, and 'in many things contradict them, I have 'thought it proper to drop this part of 'my design. It may be executed with 'more advantage, if it is at all necessary, 'after inquiring into some other powers 'of the human understanding.

'Although we have examined only the 'five senses, and the principles of the hu-'man mind which are employed about 'them, or such as have fallen in our way 'in the course of this examination, we 'shall leave the further prosecution of this 'inquiry to future deliberation. The 'powers of memory, of imagination, of 'taste, of reasoning, of moral perception, 'the will, the passions, the affections, and 'all the active powers of the soul, present 'a vast and boundless field of philosophi-'cal disquisition, which the author of this

'inquiry

'inquiry is far from thinking himſelf able 'to ſurvey with accuracy. Many authors 'of ingenuity have made excurſions into 'this vaſt territory, and have communi- 'cated uſeful obſervations, but there is 'reaſon to believe that thoſe who have 'pretended to give us a map of the whole 'have ſatisfied themſelves with a very in- 'accurate and incomplete ſurvey.'

Then ſpeaking of what Galileo and Newton have done in the natural world, he adds, 'Ambitious of following ſuch 'great examples, with unequal ſteps, alas 'and unequal force, we have attempt- 'ed an inquiry only into one little corner 'of the human mind, that corner which 'ſeems to be moſt expoſed to vulgar ob- 'ſervation, and to be moſt eaſily compre- 'hended; and yet, if we have delineated 'it juſtly, it muſt be acknowledged that 'the accounts heretofore given of it were 'very lame, and wide of the truth.'

The ſubjects our author here ſpeaks of do certainly preſent a wide field of phi- loſophical

losophical disquisition; and if so many new and important truths have occurred to our *philosopher and guide* in the examination of the five senses only, this *small corner of the human mind*, what may we not expect from his farther progress? which I hope the learned Benengeli will not fail to relate. Instinctive principles will then be as common and as cheap— but I forget the proverb—and as many distinct independent laws of nature will be found in this *microcosm* of man only, as have by others been thought necessary for the system of the universe. But what an idea must this author, and his admirers, have of the laws of nature!

Should another genius arise, and discover as many new laws in the system of *matter*, as Dr. Reid has in the system of *mind*, we should be so bewildered and confounded as hardly to retain the use of those five senses about which our author has taken so much elaborate pains. But I hope our knowledge of this part of nature is too far advanced to suffer ourselves

to

to be ſo much bewildered and puzzled, as it ſeems the inhabitants of Great-Britain and Ireland have hitherto been, with the ingenious ſpeculations of Dr. Reid.

---

# REMARKS

ON

# Dr. BEATTIE's ESSAY

ON THE

# NATURE and IMMUTABILITY

OF

# TRUTH.

THE

# INTRODUCTION.

HAVING animadverted ſo largely upon Dr. Reid's performance, I ſhall have the leſs to ſay with reſpect to that of Dr. Beattie, who adopts his general ſyſtem of *inſtinctive principles of truth*, and diſcovers too much of his ſpirit and manner, which is exceedingly deciſive, and inſolent to thoſe who think differently from himſelf; and he even exceeds Dr. Reid in throwing an odium upon thoſe whoſe ſentiments he is willing to decry, by aſcribing to them dangerous and frightful conſequences, with which they are far from being juſtly chargeable.

I believe, however, that Dr. Beattie wrote his *Eſſay on the Nature and Immutability of Truth* with the very beſt intention in the world; and that it was nothing but his zeal in the moſt excellent cauſe, that of religion, which has betrayed him into theſe raſh cenſures, and into a mode of reaſoning which I cannot help thinking to be very prejudicial to the cauſe of that very *truth* which he means to ſupport, and favouring that very *ſcepticiſm* which he imagined he was overthrowing.

I believe farther, and I moſt ſincerely rejoice in it, that Dr. Beattie's treatiſe has done a great deal of good to the cauſe of religion; and I hope it will ſtill continue to do ſo, with a great majority of thoſe who are moſt in danger of being ſeduced by the ſophiſtry of Mr. Hume, and other modern unbelievers; I mean with *ſuperficial thinkers*, who are ſatisfied with ſeeing ſuperficial objections anſwered in a lively, though a ſuperficial manner. Beſides, I do think that, in ſeveral reſpects, Dr. Beattie's ſtrictures on Mr. Hume are juſt; and therefore that they will be an uſeful antidote to the miſchief that might be apprehended from his writings.

But

But there is danger leſt other perſons, of greater penetration, finding that Dr. Beattie argues on fallacious unphiloſophical principles, ſhould reject at once, and without farther examination, all that he has built upon them. With reſpect to ſuch perſons, it may be of importance to ſhow that religion, though aſſailed from ſo many quarters as it has been of late, is under no neceſſity of taking refuge in ſuch untenable fortreſſes as Dr. Reid, Dr. Beattie, and Dr. Oſwald have provided for her; but that ſhe may ſafely face the enemy on his own ground, oppoſing argument to argument, and ſilencing ſophiſtry by rational diſcuſſion.

In this opinion I am by no means ſingular. Many judicious perſons, excellent ſcholars and divines, and whoſe metaphyſical ſyſtem is very different from mine, think Dr. Beattie's book by no means calculated to ſerve the cauſe of truth with philoſophical and thinking men; and that it will be doing ſervice to truth and religion to point out the faults and defects of it. And as I believe Dr. Beattie to be a man of candour, I doubt not but he will himself take in good part the following free animadversions. If *truth* be really our object, as it is in the titles of our books, and we be free from any improper bias, we shall rejoice in the detection of error, though it should appear to have sheltered itself under our own roofs. I am very serious when I add, that such a degree of candour and impartiality may be more especially expected of *christians*, and more especially still, of those who stand forth as champions in the cause of christianity, which is at the same time the cause of the most important truth, and of the most generous and disinterested virtue.

To preserve as much order as I well can in my remarks on Dr. Beattie's performance, I shall first consider his account of the foundation of truth, and then the several particular doctrines that he has built upon it.

SEC-

# SECTION I.

## *Of Dr.* Beattie's *account of the foundation of truth.*

OUR author adopts Dr. Reid's general idea of *common ſenſe*, as the faculty by which we perceive ſelf-evident truth, p. 37, and always conſiders it as of the nature of a peculiar kind of *inſtinct*, and very different from Locke's idea of *judgment*, in the firſt inſtance, as reſulting from comparing our ideas. This I cannot help thinking to be, theoretically ſpeaking, a very fundamental error, affecting the very *eſſence of truth*, and leading to endleſs abſurdities.

Had theſe writers aſſumed, as the elements of their common ſenſe, certain truths which are ſo plain that no man could doubt of them (without entering into the ground of our aſſent to them) their conduct would have been liable to very little objection. All that could have been ſaid would have been, that, without any neceſſity, they had made an innovation in the received uſe of a term. For no perſon ever denied that there *are* ſelf-evident truths, and that theſe muſt be aſſumed as the foundation of all our reaſoning. I never met with any perſon who did not acknowledge this, or heard of any argumentative treatiſe that did not go upon the ſuppoſition of it. The moſt rigorous reaſoners are mathematicians, and they all begin with laying down certain *axioms*, and *poſtulata*, which muſt be admitted without proof, in order to the demonſtration of every thing elſe; and therefore I am really ſurprized that Dr. Beattie, and Dr. Oſwald ſhould take ſo much pains to prove it. Had the thing been really diſputable, they have ſaid enough upon the ſubject to be quite tireſome.

But if we conſider the general tenor of their writings, it will appear that they are ſaying one thing and really doing another, talking plauſibly about the neceſſity of admitting *axioms in general*, as the foundation

dation of all reaſoning, but meaning to recommend *particular poſitions* as axioms, not as being founded on the perception of the agreement or diſagreement of any ideas, which is the great doctrine of Mr. Locke, and which makes truth to depend upon the neceſſary nature of things, to be *abſolute*, *unchangeable*, and *everlaſting;* but merely ſome unaccountable *inſtinctive perſuaſions*, depending upon the arbitrary conſtitution of our nature, which makes all truth to be a thing that is *relative* to ourſelves only, and conſequently to be infinitely vague and precarious.

This ſyſtem admits of no appeal to *reaſon*, properly conſidered, which any perſon might be at liberty to examine and diſcuſs; but, on the contrary, every man is taught to think himſelf authorized to pronounce deciſively upon every queſtion according to his preſent *feeling*, and perſuaſion; under the notion of its being ſomething original, inſtinctive, ultimate, and uncontrovertible; though, if ſtrictly analized, it might appear to be a mere prejudice, the offspring of miſtake.

This

This may appear to ſome to be, after all, a buſineſs of *metaphyſics* only, and a refinement of no real importance to mankind; but it is a miſtake that has really very ſerious and alarming conſequences; for inſtead of leading to humility, caution, and patience in the inveſtigation of truth; it neceſſarily inſpires conceit, and leads to great arrogance and inſolence with reſpect to our opponents in controverſy, as perſons defective in their conſtitution, deſtitute of common ſenſe, and therefore not to be argued with, but to be treated as ideots or madmen.

Theſe objections affect the *general ſcheme* and plan of Dr. Beattie and Dr. Oſwald. My particular objection to both theſe writers, as well as to Dr. Reid, is that they have adopted their elements of knowledge too haſtily, and that they have acquieſced in certain maxims, as ſelf-evident truths, and have treated with great inſolence and contempt all endeavours to diſprove them; though ſome of theſe maxims are ſo far from being ſelf-evident, that

in

in my opinion they are not true, but capable of a ſatisfactory refutation. At the ſame time, ſince no man can pretend to any natural right to fix the principles of faith for another, they teach unbelievers, and by their example *authorize* them, to reject the principles of religion by the ſame ſummary and ſuperficial proceſs; as what appear to them to be, at firſt ſight, too abſurd and ridiculous to be admitted as true and divine.

Though I ſhall never quarrel with any man for the mere uſe of his terms, ſince they are, in their own nature, nothing more than the arbitrary ſigns of ideas, I cannot help thinking that the inconveniencies above mentioned may attend even the calling of that faculty by which we diſcern truth by the name of *ſenſe*. By this term philoſophers in general have hitherto denominated thoſe faculties in conſequence of which we are liable to *feelings* relative to *ourſelves* only, and from which they have not pretended to draw any concluſions concerning the *nature of things*;

whereas

whereas truth is a thing not relative, but *abſolute*, and real, independent of any relation to this or that particular being, or this or that order of beings. And I think I can evidently perceive that Dr. Beattie and Dr. Oſwald have both been miſled by this new application of the term *ſenſe*; having been led by it to conſider all truth as an arbitrary thing, relative to particular beings, and even particular perſons, like the perceptions of any of our external ſenſes. In conſequence alſo of the ſame fundamental error, after having degraded the judgment to the level of the ſenſes, they naturally conſidered the ſenſes as intitled to the ſame reſpect, which had uſually been appropriated to that ſuperior faculty by which we diſtinguiſh truth.

'All that we know of truth or falſe-'hood,' ſays Dr. Beattie, p. 196, 'is that 'our conſtitution determines us in ſome 'caſes to believe, in others to diſbelieve; 'and that to us is truth which we *feel* that 'we muſt believe, and that to us is falſe-'hood which we *feel* that we muſt diſbe-'lieve.

'lieve. If, p. 209, a creature of a different 'nature from man were to ſay that ſnow 'is black and hot, I ſhould reply; it may 'poſſibly have that appearance to your 'ſenſes, but it has not that appearance to 'mine. It may therefore, in regard to 'your faculties, be true; and if ſo, it 'ought to conſtitute a part of your philo-'ſophy; but of *my* philoſophy it cannot 'conſtitute a part, becauſe, in reſpect of 'my faculties, it is falſe, being contrary 'to fact and experience.'

To me this doctrine appears to be intirely ſubverſive of all truth; ſince, ſpeaking agreeably to it, all that we can ever ſay is, that certain maxims and propoſitions appear to be true with reſpect to *ourſelves*, but how they may appear to *others* we cannot tell; and as to what they are in *themſelves*, which alone is, ſtrictly ſpeaking, the *truth*, we have no means of judging at all; for we can only ſee with our own eyes, and judge by our own faculties, or rather feelings.

If

If this be not a fair conclusion from Dr. Beattie's representation of the principles of truth and common sense I am not capable of drawing a conclusion. I am sure I do not mean to be uncandid. I hope, indeed, and believe, that he will be staggered when he attends to the unavoidable consequences of his doctrine, so very unsuitable to a discourse on the *immutability of truth*; because it is almost the very thing that he objects to Mr. Locke, whose principles he thinks *erroneous* and *dangerous*, p. 16, for speaking of one part of his philosophy he says, p. 239, 'if it be true, it would go near 'to prove that truth and virtue have at 'least nothing permanent in their nature, 'but may be as changeable as the inclinations and capacities of men.'

All the reason that our author assigns why the principle by which we judge of self-evident truth may be called a *sense* is, that such judgments are instantaneous and irresistible, like impressions made upon the mind by means of the external senses. 'The term *common sense*,' he says, p. 45, 'has,

'has, in modern times, been uſed by 'philoſophers to ſignify that power of the 'mind which perceives truth or com'mands belief, not by progreſſive argu'mentation but by an inſtantaneous, in'ſtinctive, and irreſiſtible impulſe, derived 'neither from education nor from habit, 'but from nature, acting independently 'on our will, whenever the object is pre'ſented, according to an eſtabliſhed law; 'and therefore not improperly called 'ſenſe; and acting in a ſimilar manner 'upon all, or, at leaſt, upon a great ma'jority of mankind, and therefore pro'perly called *common ſenſe*.'

But ſhould we, out of complaiſance, admit that what has hitherto been called *judgment* may be called *ſenſe*, it is making too free with the eſtabliſhed ſignification of words to call it *common ſenſe*, which in common acceptation has long been appropriated to a very different thing, viz. to that capacity for judging of common things that perſons of middling capacities are capable of.

If

If the determinations of this new principle of common ſenſe be ſo inſtantaneous, irreſiſtible, and infallible, as Dr. Reid, Dr. Beattie, and Dr. Oſwald repreſent, how can we account for all the error there is in the world? When we ſee how miſerably bewildered the bulk of mankind are, one would think that this principle of truth is like the god Baal, who when he was moſt wanted, and ought to have made a point of being preſent, to aſſiſt his worſhippers, was aſleep, or on a journey, or engaged ſome other way. See 1. Kings, xviii.

If we apply to Dr. Beattie in this great difficulty he tells us, p. 49, that 'common ſenſe may languiſh for want of exerciſe, as in the caſe of a perſon who, blinded by a falſe religion, has been all his days accuſtomed to diſtruſt his own ſentiments, and to receive his creed from the mouth of a prieſt.'

But if this languiſhing of common ſenſe reſembles the languiſhing of any other ſenſe,

ſenſe, I ſhould expect that the conſequence would be our ſeeing very dimly and obſcurely, as with a weak eye, only bearing to be uſed with great tenderneſs and caution. But though a weak eye cannot bear a ſtrong light, and only admits of faint and indiſtinct viſion, yet it exhibits all things on which it is exerciſed truly, and in their juſt proportions, or without diſtorting one thing more than another. If a man be ſo blind that he cannot ſee a houſe, neither can he ſee a tree, or any other object. I ſhould, therefore, expect that, if a man was ſo totally deprived of common ſenſe, as not to be able to diſtinguiſh truth from falſehood in one caſe, he would be equally incapable of diſtinguiſhing it in another; and therefore, that the man who ſhould put implicit faith in his prieſt would, if he wanted common ſenſe, be equally abſurd in his whole conduct, which is far from being the caſe; for in other reſpects no men think or act more rationally than the Roman Catholics. How then do the affections of this common ſenſe reſemble thoſe of the other ſenſes? The analogy appears to me to fail moſt eſſentially. It does not at all reſemble the eye, the ear, the noſe, or any other of the organs of ſenſe.

Since Dr. Beattie writes with a practical, and indeed an excellent deſign, let us conſider, for a moment, the *practical influence* of this new, and to me ſtrange doctrine. A man who finds that he thinks differently from the reſt of mankind, with reſpect to any of the principles which Dr. Beattie ſhall be pleaſed to call *primary*, and *fundamental* (ſuppoſe the doctrine of *human liberty*; or take the caſe of the poor prieſt ridden mortal above mentioned, who may with equal right conſider his own principles as fundamental) if he believes, with myſelf, and thoſe who have not yet heard of this new principle of faith, that all juſt knowledge reſults from a juſt view of things, and a comparing of his ideas, and that a habit of juſt thinking may be acquired by a courſe of obſervation and reflection duly perſiſted in; and, conſequently, that if he be in an error, it

is

is in his own power to set himself right (for that, naturally, he has as good a power of distinguishing truth from falsehood as his neighbours) a man, I say, who has these views of the nature of truth, and of the faculties by which it is perceived, is encouraged to indulge a freedom of inquiry, and to persist in his investigations, though they should prove very laborious.

Whereas, if he should have read the writers on whom I am animadverting, or Dr. Beattie only, and, in consequence of it, be persuaded that he perceives all fundamental truths by something that is of the nature of a *sense*; he may, indeed, see reason to look at any principle pretty attentively; but if, after giving this kind of attention to it, he perceives that he is not affected in that *instantaneous, instinctive*, and *irresistible* manner that Dr. Reid describes, he necessarily concludes that either it was not truth that he was contemplating, or that he is not one of that *great majority of mankind* who are endued with the faculty that is neceſſary to the perception of it. But which ever of theſe he concludes to be the caſe, he remits his attention, ſatisfied that his view of the object is conſtitutional and irremediable.

And certainly his determination would be ſufficiently countenanced by Dr. Beattie, who ſays, p. 47, that 'common ſenſe 'which, like other inſtincts, arrives at 'maturity with almoſt no care of ours, 'cannot poſſibly be taught to one who 'wants it. You may,' ſays our author, p. 47, 'make him remember a ſet of firſt 'principles, and ſay that he believes them, 'even as you may teach one born blind 'to ſpeak intelligibly of colours and light; 'but neither to the one nor to the other 'can you, by any means, communicate 'the *peculiar feeling* which accompanies 'the operation of that faculty which na- 'ture has denied him. A man defective 'in common ſenſe may acquire learning, 'he may even poſſeſs genius to a certain 'degree, but the defect of nature he ne- 'ver can ſupply. A peculiar modifica-

'tion

'tion of ſcepticiſm, or credulity, or levity, will to the end of his life diſtinguiſh him from other men.' Then, after mentioning the different *degrees* in which different men are poſſeſſed of common ſenſe, he ſays, p. 48, 'Theſe diverſities are, I think, to be referred, for the moſt part, to the original conſtitution of the mind, which it is not in the power of education to alter.'

Dr. Beattie may imagine, and I believe does, that he is ſerving *the cauſe of God and of truth* by ſuch views of things as theſe; but it appears very clearly to me, who have no pretenſions to the common ſenſe that he deſcribes, that, as far as ſpeculation can go, he is ſubverting it all.

I am aware that Dr. Beattie will reply, that this doctrine of his concerning common ſenſe is only to be applied to *firſt principles*. But who is to tell us what are firſt principles? The man who has from his infancy laboured under a miſtake, will imagine his moſt fundamental errors to be firſt principles. With a papiſt, implicit confidence in his prieſt, or holy church, which he takes for granted is the ſame thing with faith in God and the bible, acts upon his mind as *inſtantaneouſly* and *irreſiſtibly* as any of Dr. Beattie's firſt principles; and this principle in the poor papiſt cannot appear more abſurd to Dr. Beattie, than ſome of Dr. Beattie's firſt principles appear to me.

Now who is to help us in this caſe? Muſt we, in good earneſt, put the queſtion to the vote, being previouſly aſſured, by Dr. Beattie, p. 45, that a *great majority* of mankind are poſſeſſed of the true principles of common ſenſe, and therefore cannot miſtake concerning it? But I appeal from a tribunal whoſe deciſions have been ſo unſteady, and may change again; and think that nothing is ſo likely to ſerve our purpoſe, and the purpoſe of truth, as a perſuaſion the very reverſe of Dr. Beattie's, viz. that the faculty by which we perceive truth is the fartheſt

poſſible

possible from any thing that resembles a *sense*; that every misfortune we do, or may labour under, with respect to *judgment*, is naturally remediable; and consequently that it depends upon ourselves, as far as any thing of practical importance is concerned, to be as wise, judicious, and knowing, as any other person whatsoever.

Dr. Beattie seems to place the same confidence in his external senses that Dr. Reid does, which is much more than I can persuade myself to put in them; but with respect to the various instinctive principles of truth which our maker has arbitrarily annexed to them, Dr. Beattie speaks sometimes with more caution; as if he had now and then some secret distrust of them. I shall, with this view, quote what he says of the foundation of reasoning by induction and analogy.

'The mind,' he says, p. 122, 'by its 'own innate force, and in consequence 'of an irresistible and instinctive impulse, 'infers the future from the paſt, without 'the intervention of any argument. The 'ſea has ebbed and flowed twice every 'day in time paſt, therefore the ſea will 'continue to ebb and flow every day in 'time to come, is by no means a logical 'deduction of a concluſion from premiſes. 'Reaſoning from analogy,' p. 126, 'when 'traced up to its ſource, will be found in 'like manner to terminate in a certain in-'ſtinctive propenſity, implanted in us by 'our maker, which leads us to expect that 'ſimilar cauſes, in ſimilar circumſtances, 'do probably produce, or will produce, 'ſimilar effects. A child,' p. 128, 'who 'has been burned with a red hot coal is 'careful to avoid touching the flame of a 'candle. And it deſerves to be remarked 'that the judgment a child forms on theſe 'occaſions may ariſe, and often does ariſe, 'previous to education and reaſoning, 'and while experience is very limited.'

It is in this laſt clauſe that Dr. Beattie ſhows his caution, and betrays his ſuſpicion of theſe new principles. He does

not

not chuſe to ſay that children judge in this manner with *no experience at all*, which, if the judgment was properly *inſtinctive*, ought to be the caſe, (but which happens to be too notoriouſly contrary to fact) but only *when their experience is very limited.* But if they had had any experience at all, it cannot be ſaid with truth that they were without *education;* for experience is the ſchool of nature; and in this courſe of education we make much uſe of our *reaſon*, and the power of *aſſociation* is very buſily employed.

By the ſimple principle of the aſſociation of ideas, the idea of the flame of a candle is intimately aſſociated with the idea of the pain which it has occaſioned, in ſo much, that ever after they are conſidered in the cloſeſt connection, as it were the inſeparable parts of the ſame thing; ſo that whatever recals the idea of the one recals likewiſe the idea of the other, and a dread of the one cannot be ſeparated from a dread of the other.

Suppoſing

Suppoſing, therefore, that the child has an averſion to pain, and that he is maſter of thoſe actions by which it is avoided, he will mechanically, and inſtantly, draw back his hand from the near approach of a candle, without any intermediate idea whatever.

As to Dr. Reid's general principle, that *the laws of nature will continue* (with which he ſuppoſes that the mind of a child is inſpired) or, as Dr. Beattie here expreſſes it, that *ſimilar cauſes, in ſimilar circumſtances, will probably produce ſimilar effects*, as a foundation for its concluding that a candle which has burned him once will burn him again, it is not certainly at all probable that he has the leaſt notion of any ſuch thing. It is a long time before a child attains to any ſuch *general knowledge*. Particular facts are firſt diſcovered, and general propoſitions, or principles, are formed from them. But according to the hypotheſis of Dr. Reid and Dr. Beattie, the mind is, prior to any experience, either furniſhed with the

the general maxims, that there are laws of nature, and that these laws will continue, or else with a thousand particular independent maxims, comprehended under that general one. But these provisions are equally unnecessary, when the simple law of association of ideas so easily supplies the place of them both.

---

## SECTION II.

### *Of the testimony of the senses.*

THROUGH a degree of fairness and ingenuousness, for which very shrewd disputants are not always remarkable, Dr. Beattie is no less unfortunate with respect to that part of his system which relates to the *external senses*, than we have seen him to be in the instances mentioned in the last section. He speaks in general with more confidence than Dr. Reid himself does of his faith in his eyes, ears, nose, taste, and feeling (though it is possible

ſible that his writing with more ſtrength and eloquence upon this ſubject may only proceed from his having a greater command of language, and not from a ſtronger conviction of mind) but then he inadvertently ſubjoins ſuch *conceſſions*, and *exceptions*, as, in fact, overturn all his preceding doctrine, and throw us back into all our former diſtruſt of our ſenſes.

'Upon the evidence of the external 'ſenſes,' he ſays, p. 63, 'hearing, ſeeing, 'touching, taſting, and ſmelling, is 'founded all our knowledge of natural 'or material things; and therefore all 'concluſions in natural philoſophy, and 'all thoſe prudential conſiderations 'which regard the preſervation of our 'body, as it is liable to be affected by the 'ſenſible qualities of matter, muſt finally 'be reſolved into this principle, that '*things are as our ſenſes repreſent them.* 'When I touch a ſtone, I am conſcious 'of a ſenſation, or feeling in my mind, 'accompanied with an irreſiſtible belief, 'that this ſenſation is excited by the appli-

'cation

'cation of an external and hard ſubſtance
'to ſome part of my body. This belief
'as certainly accompanies the ſenſation,
'as the ſenſation accompanies the applica-
'tion of the ſtone to my organs of ſenſe.
'I am as certain,' p. 65, 'that at preſent
'I am in a houſe, and not in the open air,
'that I ſee by the light of the ſun, and
'not by the light of a candle, that I feel
'the ground hard under my feet, and
'that I lean againſt a real material
'table, as I can be of the truth of any
'geometrical axiom, or of any demon-
'ſtrated concluſion. Nay I am as cer-
'tain of all this as of my own exiſtence.
'But I cannot prove by argument that
'there is ſuch a thing as matter in the
'world, or even that I myſelf exiſt.'

All this is perfectly agreeable to the new ſyſtem, and an extremely ſhort, eaſy, and convenient one it certainly is, for thoſe who are not diſpoſed to take much pains in the inveſtigation of truth; but it is certainly not agreeable to nature and fact; and as the old proverb ſays, *Natu-*

*ram*

*ram furca licet expellas, tamen usque recurret*; so here Dr. Beattie could not help saying, p. 189, 'A distempered sense, 'as well as an impure and unequal medium, may doubtless communicate false 'sensations; but we are never imposed upon by them *in matters of consequence*.'

Now I can easily conceive how all this might have been said by Dr. Beattie very innocently, and without the least suspicion that any caviller, like myself, could possibly make any use of it to his prejudice; when, in fact, it effectually overturns his whole system of *implicit confidence in his senses*, as the sure guides to truth. For certainly, if they be capable of deceiving us *at all*, they are no more to be trusted without some guard of a different nature. The man who is under the deception has no help *from them* to undeceive himself. Thus if all mankind had jaundiced eyes, they must have been under a necessity of concluding that every object was tinged with yellow; and indeed, according to this new system, as as explained before, it would then have been ſo not in appearance only, but alſo in *reality;* nay this would have begun to be true, when only a *great majority of mankind* had their eyes thus affected.

Our author is, farther, ſo very much off his guard upon this unfortunate ſubject, as to allow that ſome of our ſenſes give us information that is contradicted by the teſtimony of others, which certainly very ill agrees with his idea of them as infallible guides to truth.

'Of magnitude,' he ſays, p. 179, 'we 'judge both by ſight and touch. With 'regard to magnitude we muſt, there'fore, believe either our ſight, or our 'touch, or both, or neither. To believe 'neither is impoſſible. If we believe 'both, we ſhall contradict ourſelves,' and at length he determines in favour of the touch. If we aſk why we believe the touch rather than the ſight, he ſays, p. 177, 'it is inſtinct, and not reaſon, that 'determines me to believe my touch.'

But

But did not he that made the ſenſe of feeling make the ſenſe of ſight alſo; and if, as our author pretends, he had deſigned that our ſenſes, *as ſuch*, ſhould give us true information concerning external objects, would he not have provided that their teſtimony ſhould have been in all reſpects perfectly conſiſtent? Beſides, it is obvious to remark, that if the eye require to be corrected by the touch, the touch may poſſibly require to be corrected by ſomething elſe. Dr. Beattie may ſay that the ſame common ſenſe that bids him believe his touch in preference to his ſight, and to correct the evidence of ſight by that of touch, aſſures him that the touch requires no correction whatever. But this can have weight only with thoſe who have faith in this ſame common ſenſe.

I ſhould be glad to aſk Dr. Beattie, and others who admit it as a maxim, that *things are as their ſenſes repreſent them to be*, what a man of common ſenſe, and altogether without experience (which indeed

deed can hardly be the caſe in fact) would ſay upon looking at a ſtraight ſtick held obliquely, with half of it under water. Would he not be poſitive that it was bent in the middle; and would he not have the plain teſtimony of his eyes for it? If you ſhould take the ſtick out of the water, and bid him look at it again, and handle it, would he not aſſert the very reverſe of Dr. Beattie's maxim, viz. that his eyes had *impoſed* upon him, and that *the thing was not as his ſenſes had repreſented it?*

Do not the bulk of mankind believe that the earth is at reſt, and that the ſun, moon, and ſtars have a diurnal revolution; and have they not the teſtimony of their ſenſes for it? They certainly *think* ſo. They alſo all believe (as Dr. Reid himſelf pretends to believe with them) that colour is a property of bodies, and yet are eaſily convinced that it is a miſtake.

If, after all, it really be a dictate of this new common ſenſe, that, notwithſtanding all this, things ſtill are as our ſenſes repreſent them to be, I think that in theſe caſes our common ſenſe is in league with our other ſenſes to impoſe upon us, and therefore that we are juſtified in excluding it, as well as them, from being the teſt of truth.

---

## SECTION III.

*Dr.* Beattie's *view of* Berkley's *theory.*

IT is curious to obſerve how much our acquaintance both with truth and error reſembles the introduction of the fox to the lion, in the fable of Eſop. We grow bolder by degrees, and each encourages his neighbour to go a few ſteps farther than himſelf.

The principles both of Dr. Reid and Dr. Beattie lead them to reject Berkley's hypotheſis. Indeed, their whole ſcheme appears to me to have been, in a great meaſure

measure, suggested by it; but Dr. Beattie rises greatly upon Dr. Reid in his tone and emphasis upon this occasion. If Dr. Reid conquered and slew his adversary, Dr. Beattie not only conquers, and puts him to death a second time, but tramples upon him. Dr. Reid did not vanquish him till after a pretty hard combat, in which some skill and dexterity in the use of his weapons was requisite; but Dr. Beattie does it at once, without giving him an opportunity of drawing in his own defence. Hear his own account of their different modes of conducting this controversy.

'Though it be absurd,' says Dr. Beattie, p. 290, 'to attempt a proof of what is 'self-evident, it is manly and meritorious 'to confute the objections that sophistry 'may urge against it. This, with respect 'to the subject in question, has been done 'in a decisive and masterly manner by 'Dr. Reid, who proves that the reasonings of Berkley, and others, concerning 'primary and secondary qualities owe all

'their ſtrength to the ambiguity of words."
This, then, is the *manly* and *meritorious* conduct of Dr. Reid; but being only of relative uſe and importance, and *abſurd in itſelf*, our author takes a different ground; which he immediately deſcribes. 'I have proved that though this fundamental error had never been detected, 'the philoſophy of Berkley is, in its own 'nature, abſurd, becauſe it ſuppoſes the 'original principles of common ſenſe 'controvertible and fallacious; a ſuppoſition repugnant to the genius of the 'true' (alias the *new*) 'philoſophy, and 'which leads to univerſal credulity, or 'univerſal ſcepticiſm, and conſequently 'to the ſubverſion of knowledge and vir- 'tue, and'—but firſt gueſs reader, if you can, what follows—'the extermination of 'the human ſpecies.' He even fixes the time, very nearly, in which this calamitous event would take place.

Deſcribing what he imagined would follow if all mankind ſhould, in one inſtant, be made to believe that matter has

no

no exiſtence, he ſays, p. 281, 'Doubtleſs 'this cataſtrophe would, according to our 'metaphyſicians, throw a wonderful light 'on all the parts of knowledge. I pre- 'tend not even to gueſs at the number, 'extent, or quality, of the aſtoniſhing diſ- 'coveries that would then ſtart forth into 'view. But of this I am certain, that, in '*leſs than a month* after, there could not, 'without another miracle, be one human 'creature alive on the face of the earth.'

Dr. Reid fairly encounters his enemy, vanquiſhes, ſlays, and buries him, all in their proper order; but Dr. Beattie begins at once with the laſt act of burying, without troubling himſelf whether he be dead or alive, thinking the act of burying will ſuffice for all. This is that curious and ſummary proceſs which Dr. Oſwald is taking to rid the world of all dangerous errors in religion. Without giving himſelf the unneceſſary trouble to argue the matter, except for his own amuſement, and that of his readers, he only throws himſelf back in his chair, ſhuts his eyes, ſees them to be abſurd, and the deluſion vaniſhes. This is indeed fighting with the ſpear of Ithuriel, at the touch of which all impoſture vaniſhes *.

I ſhall quote one paſſage more from Dr. Beattie on this ſubject, in which he expreſſes the nature and fullneſs of his perſuaſion concerning the reality of the material world, in a manner that is peculiarly emphatical, and therefore muſt be very ſatisfactory to men of *taſte*, who can feel the beauties of fine writing. 'That matter has a real, ſeparate, and 'independent exiſtence,' p. 261, 'is be-'lieved, not becauſe it can be proved by 'argument, but becauſe the conſtitution

* The paſſage in Dr. Oſwald, to which I here allude, is ſo very curious, that I think my reader will not be diſpleaſed to ſee it quoted in a note on this part of my remarks on Dr. Beattie, though he will find it quoted again in its proper place. 'A real believer,' p. 255, 'will not deſpiſe 'the well-meant labours of thoſe who have endeavoured to 'demonſtrate the primary truths by reducing their oppo-'ſites to abſurdity; but knows, that, without their help, 'he can, *by a ſingle thought*, reduce thoſe chimeras to the 'groſſeſt of all abſurdities, namely, to nonſenſe.'

'of

'of our nature is ſuch, that we *muſt* believe it. There is here the ſame ground of belief, that there is in the following propoſitions. I exiſt; whatever is is; two and two make four. It is abſurd, nay it is impoſſible to believe the contrary.' Accordingly, he ſays, 'I have known many who could not anſwer Berkley's arguments, I never knew one who believed his doctrine.'

I find, however, that I have travelled a little farther than Dr. Beattie, for I have met with a very ingenious man who maintained Berkley's doctrine with great ſeriouſneſs, and I have known others who have eſpouſed the ſame opinion. But perhaps Dr. Beattie may have the indulgence of the Welch jury I have heard of, who would not believe a man who confeſſed himſelf to be guilty, and fairly acquitted him.

My friend and I uſed to debate this ſubject, but for want of being acquainted with the principles of Meſſrs. Reid, Beattie, and

Oſwald, I was glad to plead for the exiſtence of the material world only as the moſt probable hypotheſis to account for appearances, and never thought of there being the ſame kind of evidence for it, as of two and two being equal to four. Had I been acquainted with theſe new principles, I might have ſaved myſelf a great deal of trouble; but I am apprehenſive that I ſhould hardly have eſcaped a great deal of *ridicule ;* and we ought not to forget that ridicule has been deemed the *teſt of truth* as well as this new common ſenſe. I think with equal reaſon, and I flatter myſelf that the reign of this new uſurper will not be much longer than that of his predeceſſor, to whom he is very nearly related.

In this ſome may think that I only mean to be jocular, but really I am ſerious. Why was *ridicule* ever thought to be the teſt of truth, but becauſe the things at which we can laugh were ſuppoſed to be ſo abſurd, that their falſehood was ſelf-evident; ſo that there was no occa-

ſion

ſion to examine any farther? We were ſuppoſed to *feel* them to be falſe; and what is a *feeling* but the affection of a *ſenſe?* In reality, therefore, this new doctrine of common ſenſe being the ſtandard of truth is no other than ridicule being the ſtandard of truth. The words are different, but not the things. I ſhould be glad to ſee ſo acute a metaphyſician as Dr. Reid, ſo fine a writer as Dr. Beattie, and, to adopt Dr. Beattie's compliment, ſo *elegant an author* as Dr. Oſwald, ſeparately employed to aſcertain the preciſe difference between theſe two ſchemes.

In my opinion the chief difference, beſides what I ſaid above, conſiſts in this, that the one may be called the *ſenſe of truth*, and the other the *ſenſe of falſehood*. There is alſo ſome doubt whether Shafteſbury was really in earneſt in propoſing ridicule as the teſt of truth. Many think that he never could be ſo abſurd. Whereas there can be no doubt but that this triumvirate of authors are perfectly ſerious. There is, however, another difference that will ſtrongly

ſtrongly recommend the claims of common ſenſe in preference to thoſe of ridicule, which is, that *this* was advanced in ſupport of infidelity, but *that* in ſupport of religion. But I ſhould think that the greater weight we have to ſupport, the ſtronger buttreſſes we ſhould uſe.

In remarking upon Dr. Reid, I pointed out the inconcluſiveneſs of the conſequences he drew from Berkley's hypotheſis. Dr. Beattie ſays the ſame things after him, but with conſiderable improvements in point of diction and energy, and with an air of much greater ſeriouſneſs with reſpect to *religion,* which appears to me to have nothing to do in the buſineſs. I do not wonder, however, at Dr. Beattie's zeal in the caſe, when he imagined that ſo much depended upon it, any more than I do at Don Quixote's heroic enthuſiaſm, when he miſtook inns for caſtles, a flock of ſheep for an army, and a barber's baſon for Mambrino's helmet.

'Sure,'

'Sure,' ſays our author, p. 283, 'the 'laws of nature are not ſuch trifles as that 'it muſt be a matter of perfect indifference 'whether we act or think agreeable to 'them or no.' I think if I had not apprized my reader of it before hand, he would not have gueſſed that, in this ſolemn ſentence, our author had nothing in view but this ſame innocent theory of Berkley; and eſpecially if he had not ſeen, in the preceding quotation, that the very *extermination of the human ſpecies* is the conſequence of this ſame ſcheme; which appears to me to be as complete raving as any thing in Don Quixote himſelf.

Our author farther ſays, p. 289, 'Berk'ley's doctrine is ſubverſive of man's moſt 'important intereſts, as a moral, intelli'gent, and percipient being. I doubt 'not,' ſays he, ib. 'but it may have over'caſt many of his days with a gloom, 'which neither the approbation of his 'conſcience, nor the natural ſerenity of 'his temper could intirely diſſipate.'

Now

Now I can ſee no difficulty in conceiving that I myſelf might have adopted this opinion, and yet have been very eaſy, chearful, virtuous, religious, and happy, in the full expectation of a reſtoration to a future life, as real as that which I enjoy at preſent, and in circumſtances infinitely ſuperior. In ſo very different lights do we ſometimes ſee the ſame thing, though we are all, at leaſt we all *think* ourſelves, poſſeſſed of this ſame infallible ſtandard of truth, viz. *common ſenſe.*

## SECTION IV.

*Dr.* Beattie's *account of the ſource of* moral obligation, *and of the fundamental principles of religion.*

HITHERTO I muſt acknowledge that I have not always been able to reſiſt the temptation to divert myſelf with my author's Quixotiſm. For, ſerious as he himſelf has been, his adventures have ſometimes appeared laughable enough to me. But I muſt now begin to be a little more ſerious, becauſe I apprehend the conſequences are ſo. For our author, after having made his common ſenſe the *teſt of truth,* proceeds to make it the ſtandard of *moral obligation,* expreſsly excluding all reaſoning upon the ſubject.

'They,' ſays Dr. Beattie, p. 74, meaning mankind, 'believe a certain mode of 'conduct to be incumbent upon them in 'certain circumſtances, becauſe a notion 'of duty ariſes in their mind when they

con-

'contemplate that conduct in relation to 'those circumstances. I ought to be 'grateful for a favour received. Why? 'because my conscience tells me so. How 'do you know that you ought to do that 'of which your conscience enjoins the 'performance? I can give no further 'reason for it but I *feel* that such is my 'duty. Here the investigation must stop; 'or if carried a little farther, it must re-'turn to this point. I know that I ought 'to do what my conscience enjoins be-'cause God is the author of my constitu-'tion, and I obey his will when I act ac-'cording to the principles of my constitu-'tion. Why do you obey the will of 'God? Because it is my duty. How 'know you that? Because my conscience 'tells me so, &c.

In any other case, therefore, if a man *feels* that any thing is his duty, or, which is the same thing with respect to himself, if he *thinks* he feels it, he has no occasion to trouble himself with examining into the ground of that feeling. He must follow

follow it without hesitation, or reserve. So that even the poor priest-ridden mortal above mentioned will be justified, if, at the command of his ghostly superior, he murders his heretical neighbour; for had he gone the round of the self examination described by Dr. Beattie, it would have been like travelling round the world for nothing but to come to the same place from which he set out, viz. *so my conscience dictates.*

Judging in the first and last instance by mere *feeling*, it is impossible to distinguish the injunctions of a *well-informed* from those of an *ill-informed* conscience. Many, I doubt not, have felt as real remorse upon the omission of a superstitious ceremony, and have been as unhappy in consequence of it, as they have ever been for the neglect of the most important moral duty. As, on the other hand, they have felt as real satisfaction after confessing to a priest, and having received his absolution, as others have felt from the consciousness of genuine repentance, or of a well ſpent life. Yea ſome, I am perſuaded, have felt as perfectly eaſy at a Portugueſe *act of faith*, as if they had been *glorifying God* in any other manner.

Not content with this, Dr. Beattie ſcruples not to reſt all the future hopes and expectations of man, as derived from religion, on the foundation of this ſame principle of common ſenſe. 'Scep-'tics,' ſays Dr. Beattie, p. 113, 'may 'wrangle, and mockers may blaſpheme; 'but the pious man knows, by evidence 'too ſublime for their comprehenſion, 'that his affections are not miſplaced, 'and that his hopes ſhall not be diſap-'pointed; by evidence which to every 'ſound mind is fully ſatisfactory, but 'which to the humble and tender hearted 'is altogether overwhelming, irreſiſtible, 'and divine.'

With whatever feelings Dr. Beattie might compoſe this paragraph, it ſtrikes me as containing matter that is exceedingly dangerous and alarming; ſetting aſide

aside all reasoning about the fundamental principles of religion, and making way for all the extravagancies of credulity, enthusiasm, and mysticism.

The *plenary persuasion* that our religious *affections are not misplaced*, and that our *hopes shall not be disappointed*, evidently supposes the belief of the being, the perfections, and moral attributes of God, and a state of future retribution; and what *kind* of evidence has Dr. Beattie spoken of as *overwhelming*, and *irresistible*, but this of common sense? the effects of which he always describes in that style, and to which he had before applied those very epithets, and others of a similar import. And yet this common sense appears to me, and to others, who seem to be in our sober senses, to be very insufficient for this purpose; though Dr. Oswald has attempted to prove at large, and in detail, all the particulars which Dr. Beattie only asserts in gross. But I am afraid that, after all his pious pains, the evidence will be found to be what Dr.

 Beattie

Beattie here ſays of it, *too ſublime for our comprehenſion.*

That our author imagined he had ſufficiently eſtabliſhed ſome very important religious and practical principles, is evident from what he ſays in the concluſion of his work, where he is reciting his achievements in it. 'That the human 'ſoul is a real and permanent ſubſtance,' he ſays, p. 491, 'that God is infinitely 'wiſe and good, that virtue and vice are 'eſſentially different, that there is ſuch a 'thing as truth, and that man, in many 'caſes, is capable of diſcovering it, are 'ſome of the principles which this book 'is intended to vindicate from the ob'jections of ſcepticiſm.

Now I do not recollect, after reading Dr. Beattie's book through (with how much attention and care let the reader judge) that he has attempted a demonſtration of the human ſoul being a rational and permanent ſubſtance, of the infinite wiſdom and goodneſs of God, that virtue and

and vice are eſſentially different, &c. by any proper medium of proof whatever; but only, if he has proved them at all, by an appeal to this principle of common ſenſe, which is ſaid to aſſure us, *without reaſoning*, that ſuch and ſuch doctrines are true.

Alſo, though Dr. Beattie has not taken the ſame large field of argument that Dr. Oſwald has done, thinking probably that, after him, it was unneceſſary, yet he quotes from him with reſpect, and no doubt with intire approbation (or why did he quote him at all?) a paſſage in which he not only aſſerts the propriety of defending primary truths on the ſole authority of common ſenſe, but vindicates the doing of it with a peculiar *emphaſis*, and without much delicacy. And I have already ſhewn in what an extenſive ſenſe Dr. Oſwald conſiders the primary truths of religion, a ſenſe with which Dr. Beattie could not be unacquainted.

Dr. Beattie's quotation, in vindication of his vehemence of expreſſion in this treatiſe, is as follows, p. 512. 'There 'is no ſatisfying the demands of falſe 'delicacy, ſays an elegant and pious au-'thor, becauſe they are not regulated by 'any fixed ſtandard. But a man of can-'dour and judgment will allow that the 'baſhful timidity, practiſed by thoſe who 'put themſelves on a level with the ad-'verſaries of religion, would ill become 'one who, declining all diſputes, aſſerts 'primary truths on the authority of com-'mon ſenſe; and that whoever pleads 'the cauſe of religion in this way has a 'right to aſſume a firmer tone, and to 'pronounce with a more deciſive air, not 'upon the ſtrength of his own judgment, 'but on the reverence due from all man-'kind to the tribunal to which he appeals. '*Oſwald's appeal in behalf of religion*, 'p. 14.' Theſe gentlemen, therefore, having diſcarded all pretences to *reaſoning*, think themſelves juſtified in diſcarding all *good manners*, and in aſ-

ſuming

ſuming an arrogance and inſolence which does not become us poor reaſoners. A happy privilege truly!

From theſe circumſtances it appears to me to be impoſſible not to conclude, that Dr. Beattie approved, in the main, of what Dr. Oſwald had written. Indeed, writing upon this ſubject, and mentioning him at all, it behoved him to have guarded his readers againſt his dangerous extravagancies, if he had not gone the ſame lengths himſelf. His candid letter to me, however, which the reader will find at the end of this book, makes me conclude, that he does not *now* approve of Dr. Oſwald's writings; and I hope that, after more reflection, he will acknowledge that he has given his abſurd and dangerous principles too much countenance by what he has written himſelf.

## SECTION V.

*Dr.* Beattie's *view of the doctrine of* necessity.

AFTER the very severe and injurious treatment that Bishop Berkley's amusing theory has met with, it cannot be expected that the doctrine of *necessity*, which, like many other very good things, has had the misfortune to fall into the hands of some unbelievers, should escape Dr. Beattie's censure; especially as, like other great truths, removed from the conception of the vulgar (as that of the revolution of the earth upon its axis) it necessarily stands exposed to some plausible, but superficial, objections. There is, at the bottom, however, something so ingenuous in Dr. Beattie, that, notwithstanding the vehemence of his assertions, he has not been able to conceal evident marks of the impression that has been upon him by the arguments of the Necessarians. These, I doubt not, have had

had no ſmall influence in determining him to ſhut his eyes ſo obſtinately, to diſclaim all *argument* upon the ſubject, and to take refuge in his moſt convenient and never failing principle of *common ſenſe*.

Both the thorough ſatisfaction that Dr. Beattie has in his own principles, and the manner in which he attained and preſerves that ſatisfaction, notwithſtanding the *unanſwerable arguments* (as he can hardly help acknowledging) of the Neceſſarians, may be ſeen in the following quotations, which I can read and tranſcribe without feeling myſelf more offended than I ſhould be at hearing any perſon aſſert his full conviction of *the earth ſtanding ſtill*; being fully ſatisfied with the evidence that I have of the very ſuperficial grounds on which his opinion has been formed.

'My intention,' p. 295, 'is to treat 'the doctrine of neceſſity as I have 'treated that of non-exiſtence of matter, 'by inquiring whether the one be not, as 'well as the other, contrary to common 'sense, and therefore absurd. Both doc-'trines,' p. 360, 'are repugnant to the 'general belief of mankind, both, not-'withstanding all the efforts of the subtlest 'sophistry, are still incredible; both are 'so contrary to nature, and to the condi-'tion of human beings, that they can-'not be carried into practice, and so con-'trary to true philosophy, that they can-'not be admitted into science; without 'bringing scepticism along with them, 'and rendering questionable the plainest 'principles of moral truth, and the very 'distinction between truth and falsehood. 'In a word, we have proved that com-'mon sense, as it teaches us to believe, 'and be assured of the existence of mat-'ter, doth also teach us to believe, and be 'assured, that man is a free agent. My 'liberty, in these instances,' p. 295, 'I can-'not prove by argument, but there is not 'a truth in geometry of which I am more 'certain.' Speaking of the same thing, he says, p. 311, 'Some philosophers 'want

'want to prove what I know by inſtinct 'to be unqueſtionably certain. I am as 'conſcious,' p. 70, 'that ſome actions 'are in my power, and that others are 'not, &c. as I am of my own exiſtence.'

I have no occaſion to enter into a diſcuſſion of this queſtion with Dr. Beattie. Indeed, I am precluded from doing it; for what can it avail to argue with a man who declares that he will neither argue himſelf, nor hear the arguments of others upon the ſubject? But to anſwer this very pertinacious believer, in ſomething of his own way, I will tell him that, if I were to take my choice of any metaphyſical queſtion, to defend it againſt all oppugners, it ſhould be this very abſurd and obnoxious doctrine of *neceſſity*, of the falſehood of which our author is as certain as he is of his own exiſtence. There is no truth of which I have leſs doubt, and of the grounds of which I am more fully ſatisfied; and I am likewiſe fully perſuaded, not only of the perfect *innocence*, but alſo of the *happy moral influence* of

it.

it. Indeed, there is no abſurdity more glaring to my underſtanding than the notion of *philoſophical liberty*; and (judging as Dr. Beattie does of Berkley's theory) of more dangerous conſequence. But I have long learned to entertain no great dread of opinions theoretically dangerous, and to repeat what I have ſaid upon a former occaſion, 'Notwithſtanding ſome ſects do, in words, ſubvert the 'foundations of all virtue, they have always ſome *ſalvo* whereby they preſerve 'a regard to it, and in reality enforce it. 'Such a foundation has the God of nature laid for the practice of virtue in 'our hearts, that it is hardly in the power 'of any error in our heads to eraſe it.' *Diſcourſe on the Lord's Supper, third edition, p.* 107.

What could lead Dr. Beattie to quote Dr. Hartley upon the ſubject I cannot tell, as he does not propoſe to enter into any diſcuſſion of the queſtion, except it was to take an opportunity of contradicting him in his appeal to experience with relation to it. 'In all my experience,' ſays

ſays he, p. 333, 'I have never been con-
'ſcious of any ſuch neceſſity as the au-
'thor (Dr. Hartley) ſpeaks of.' But ſo very little attention did Dr. Beattie give to any thing like *reaſoning* on this ſubject, or even neceſſary explanations of it, that though Dr. Hartley, in the very paſſage that Dr. Beattie quotes from him, gives a very accurate ſtate of the queſtion, defining philoſophical liberty to be *a power of doing different things, the motives, or previous circumſtances, remaining preciſely the ſame,* all that our author ſays upon the ſubject ſhows that the liberty which he contends for is *the power of doing what we pleaſe, or will,* which Dr. Hartley is far from denying.

It makes me ſmile, and I am confident it muſt make others ſmile, who ſhall read both theſe writers, to find Dr. Beattie calling Dr. Hartley *a fanciful author.* To judge by the ſtyle and manner of the two writers, I think any indifferent perſon would ſee that ſerious and diſpaſſionate argument was with Dr. Hartley, and *fancy* and *imagination* wholly with Dr. Beattie.

There

There is ſomething very ſingular in the *manner* in which Dr. Beattie treats this ſubject of neceſſity; firſt diſclaiming all reaſoning about it, then, from his natural ingenuouſneſs, not being able intirely to ſatisfy himſelf with this conduct, half hinting at ſome objections, and ſubjoining ſome half anſwers to them; then acknowledging that the arguments on both ſides *come at laſt to appear unanſwerable*, p. 362, and ſo reverting to his common ſenſe again; juſt as he did in his account of the foundation of moral obligation, in which he both began and ended with an appeal to the ſame common ſenſe.

Among other things, our author gently touches upon the objection to the contingency of human actions from the doctrine of the *divine preſcience*. In anſwer to which, or rather in *deſcanting* upon which (thinking I ſuppoſe, to chuſe the leſs of two evils) he ſeems to make no great difficulty of rejecting that moſt eſſential prerogative of the divine nature, though nothing can be

more

more fully aſcertained by independent evidence from revelation, rather than give up his darling hypotheſis of human liberty; ſatisfying himſelf with obſerving, p. 352, that 'it implies no reflection on 'the divine power, that it cannot perform 'impoſſibilities.' In the very ſame manner he might make himſelf perfectly eaſy if his hypotheſis ſhould compel him to deny any other of the attributes of God, or even his very being, for what reflection is it upon any perſon that things impoſſible cannot be. Thus our author, in the blind rage of diſputation, heſitates not to deprive the ever bleſſed God of that very attribute by which, in the books of ſcripture, he expreſsly diſtinguiſhes himſelf from all falſe Gods, and than which nothing can be more eſſentially neceſſary to the government of the univerſe, rather than relinquiſh his fond claim to the fancied privilege of *ſelf-determination*; a claim which appears to me to be juſt as abſurd as that of *ſelf-exiſtence*, and which could not poſſibly do him any good if he had it.

Terrified,

Terrified, however, as I am willing to suppose (though he does not express any such thing, as he seems to be ready, upon any emergency, with all the *sang-froid* in the world, to strike from his creed the doctrine of the divine prescience) at this consequence of his system, he thinks, with those who maintain the doctrine of a *trinity* of persons in the unity of the divine essence, and with those who assert the doctrine of *transubstantiation*, to shelter himself in the *obscurity* of his subject; saying, p. 353, that 'we cannot 'comprehend the manner in which the 'divine being operates.' But this refuge is equally untenable in all the cases, because the things themselves are, in their own nature, impossible, and imply a contradiction. I might just as well say that, though to us, whose understandings are so limited, *two* and *two* appear to make no more than *four;* yet in the divine mind, the comprehension of which is infinite, into which, however, we cannot look, and concerning which it is impossible,

and

and even dangerous to form conjectures, they may make *five*.

Were I possessed of Dr. Beattie's talent of declamation, and had as little scruple to make use of it, what might I not say of the absurdity of this way of talking, and of the horrible immoral consequences of denying the fore-knowledge of God? I should soon make our author and all his adherents as black as atheists. The very admission of so untractable a principle as *contingency* into the universe would be no better than admitting the Manichean doctrine of an *independent evil principle;* nay it would be really of worse consequence; for the one might be controlled, but the other could not. But I thank God my principles are more generous, and I am as far from ascribing to Dr. Beattie all the real consequences of his doctrine, (which, if, he could see with my eyes, I believe he would reprobate as heartily as I do myself) as I am from admitting his injurious imputations with respect to mine.

Not-

Notwithstanding Dr. Beattie, confiding in the solidity of his own judgment, strengthened by the sanction of *a great majority of mankind*, is pleased to call Dr. Hartley a *fanciful author*, he does vouchsafe, at the same time, to call him *an ingenious and worthy one*, which, considering the horrid consequences he deduces from his principles, must argue a great deal of candour. But, indeed, I think it absolutely impossible for any person to read his *Observations on man*, and not lay down the book with the fullest conviction both of the amazing comprehensiveness and strength of his mind (to which the trifling epithet of *ingenious* is very inadequate) and of the piety, benevolence and rectitude of his heart. All who were acquainted with him join their testimony to this internal evidence from his writings.

Without, however, attempting to account for this, or any facts of the same kind, our author takes it for granted, p. 473, 351, that the doctrine of necessity is incon-

inconſiſtent with the firſt principles of natural religion. After enumerating a number of abſurd and atheiſtical tenets, he ſums up the whole with ſaying, p. 317 ——' and now the liberty of the human ' will is queſtioned and debated. What ' could we expect but that it ſhould ſhare ' the ſame fate?' ' To believe,' ſays he, p. 355, ' that the dictates of conſcience ' are falſe, unreaſonable, or inſignificant, ' is one certain effect of my becoming a ' fataliſt, or even ſceptical with regard to ' moral liberty.' If I could think that this would be the conſequence, I ſhould be very ſorry to hear of Dr. Beattie's changing his ſentiments on this ſubject; but we know very little of our own hearts, and what we ſhould think, feel, or do, in very new ſituations. For my own part, I doubt not but that this very change of opinion which he dreads ſo much (if it be not too late for him to bear the ſhock that ſo total a revolution in his ſyſtem of thinking would occaſion) would bear a very favourable aſpect on his virtue, and even make him a better man than he is at

 preſent;

present; though, by all accounts, he is a very good one.

As to the hackneyed objection to the doctrine of necessity, from its being inconsistent with the idea of virtue and vice, as implying praise and blame, it may be fully retorted upon its opponents. For as to their boasted *self-determining power* (were the thing possible in itself, and did not imply an absurdity) by which they pretend to have a power of acting independently of every thing that comes under the description of *motive*, I scruple not to say, that it is as foreign to every idea of virtue or vice, praise or blame, as the grossest kind of mechanism, that the most blundering writer in defence of liberty ever ascribed to the advocates for moral necessity.

It is true that, strictly speaking, the doctrine of necessity would oblige a man to depart from the common *language* in speaking of human actions; but this makes no change with respect to his *conduct*.

The

The very ſame is the caſe with reſpect to the doctrine of the *ſun ſtanding ſtill.* Philoſophers uſe the language of the vulgar with reſpect to this ſubject, and even *think* with them too, except in their cloſets, and when they are explicitly attending to it. Copernicus and Newton themſelves, I will venture to ſay, not only talked of the ſun riſing and ſetting, but, *in their ordinary conceptions,* had the very ſame ideas that a common farmer annexes to thoſe words. So alſo it is impoſſible that, with reſpect to common life, a neceſſarian ſhould have any other ideas to the words praiſe and blame (which however are equally foreign to both the ſchemes of liberty and neceſſity, philoſophically and ſtrictly conſidered) than other people have, and he will be influenced as much by them. And as to the different views that he will be able to take of theſe things in *contemplation,* they appear to me only to remove virtue from one foundation to place it upon another, much broader and firmer. Our conduct depends not upon what we *think* our conſtitution to be, but upon what it really *is*. But upon this ſubject I refer to Dr. Hartley, both for argument, and example.

Upon this, as upon a former occaſion, I cannot help obſerving what different company I and Dr. Beattie have kept. 'I 'have found,' ſays he, p. 344, 'all the 'impartial, the moſt ſagacious, and wor-'thy part of mankind, enemies to fatality 'in their hearts.' On the contrary, a conſiderable majority of my acquaintance, men of whoſe underſtanding and hearts not myſelf only, but all who know them, have the higheſt opinion, have been, and are, confirmed neceſſarians.

For my own part, if I might be allowed to follow Dr. Beattie's example, in appealing to my own experience, I would tell him, that I embraced the doctrine of neceſſity from the time that I firſt ſtudied the ſubject; I have been a firm believer of it ever ſince, without having ever entertained the leaſt ſuſpicion of there being any fallacy belonging to it; I meditate

I meditate frequently upon it, and yet every confideration of it, and every view of things fuggefted by it, appears to me to give an elevation to the fentiments, the moft exalted conceptions of the great author of nature, and of the excellence and perfection of his works and defigns, the greateft purity and fervor to our virtue, the moft unbounded benevolence to our fellow creatures, the moft ardent zeal to ferve them, and the moft unreferved and joyful confidence in divine providence, with refpect to all things, paft, prefent, and to come.

In fhort, I have no conception that the man whofe mind is capable of entertaining, and duly contemplating what is called the doctrine of neceffity, and its genuine confequences, as unfolded by Dr. Hartley, can be a bad man; nay that he can be other than an extraordinary good one. I am confident that I fhall improve myfelf continually by frequent and *fteady* views of this fubject, and fuch as are connected with it, and by being actuated by them more than I have been. It is true that I had the unspeakable happiness of a very strict and religious education; but notwithstanding this, had the doctrine of necessity, in reality, any immoral tendency, I am positive it would have done me an irreparable injury at the time that I adopted it.

Let Dr. Beattie reflect upon these things with the candour that I am willing to think is natural to him, and I doubt not he will feel himself disposed to unsay some of the harsh things that have dropped from him on this subject.

That my reader may enjoy the pleasure of *contrast* in a higher degree, I shall subjoin to this section a few extracts from Mr. Jonathan Edwards, in which he expresses his opinion of the unfavourable tendency of the doctrine of philosophical liberty, which he calls the *Arminian* doctrine, with respect to virtue and religion, &c. in his *Treatise on free will;* which I had not read till after the whole of of this book, and even the preface, except the paragraph relating to it, was transcribed for the press.

'Arminian principles and notions,' p. 267, 'when fairly examined, and 'pursued in their demonstrable consequences, do evidently shut all virtue 'out of the world, and make it impossible that there should ever be any 'such thing, in any case, or that any such 'thing should ever be conceived of. For 'by these principles the very notion of 'virtue or vice implies absurdity and 'contradiction."

'A moral necessity of men's actions,' p. 16, Appendix, 'is not at all inconsistent with any liberty that any creature 'has, or can have, as a free, accountable, 'moral agent, and subject of moral go-'vernment. This moral necessity is so 'far from being inconsistent with praise 'and blame, and the benefit and use of 'men's own care and labour, that, on the 'contrary, it implies the very ground and 'reason why men's actions are to be 'ascribed to them as their own, in that 'manner as to infer desert, praise and 'blame, approbation and remorse of con-'science, reward and punishment; and it 'establishes the moral system of the uni-'verse, and God's moral government, in 'every respect, with the proper use of 'motives, exhortations, commands, coun-'cils, promises and threatnings, and the 'use and benefit of endeavours, care and 'industry; and therefore there is no need 'that the strict philosophic truth should 'be at all concealed from men. So far 'from this, the truth in this matter is of 'vast importance, and extremely need-'ful to be known, and the more con-'stantly it is in view the better.'

'The moral necessity of men's actions,' p. 7. 'is requisite to the being of virtue 'and vice, or any thing praise-worthy or 'culpable; and the liberty of indifference, 'and contingence, which is advanced in 'opposition to that necessity, is incon-'sistent with the being of these.—If we 'pursue

'pursue these principles,' p. 258, 'we shall 'find that virtue and vice are wholly ex'cluded out of the world, and that there 'never was, or ever can be, any such 'thing as one or the other, either in God, 'angels, or men.'

'The doctrine of necessity,' p. 386, 'which supposes a necessary connection 'of all events, on some antecedent ground 'and reason of their existence, is the only 'medium we have to prove the being of 'God. And the contrary doctrine of 'contingence, which certainly implies, or 'infers, that events may come into ex'istence, or begin to be, without de'pendence on any thing foregoing, as 'their cause, ground, or reason, takes 'away all proof of the being of God.'

'It is so far from being true,' p. 15, 'that our minds are naturally possessed 'with a notion of such liberty as this, (so 'strongly that it is impossible to root it 'out) that, indeed, men have no such 'notion of liberty at all, and it is utterly

'impossible,

'impoſſible, by any means whatſoever, 'to implant or introduce ſuch a notion 'into the mind.—The greateſt and moſt 'learned advocates themſelves for liberty 'of indifference and ſelf-determination 'have no ſuch notion; and indeed they 'mean ſomething wholly inconſiſtent 'with, and directly ſubverſive of, what 'they ſtrenuouſly affirm, and earneſtly 'contend for.'

'All the Arminians on earth,' p. 411, 'might be challenged, without arrogance, 'to make theſe principles of theirs con- 'ſiſtent with common ſenſe, yea and per- 'haps to produce any doctrine ever em- 'braced by the blindeſt bigot of the 'church of Rome, or the moſt ignorant 'Muſſulman, or extravagant enthuſiaſt, 'that might be reduced to more, and 'more demonſtrable inconſiſtencies and 'repugnancies to common ſenſe, and to 'themſelves; though their inconſiſtencies 'may not, indeed, lie ſo deep, or be ſo 'artfully vailed by a deceitful ambiguity of 'of words, and an indeterminate signi-'fication of phrases.'

How very different is the *common sense* of Mr. Edwards from the common sense of Dr. Beattie! How uniform and infallible is this guide to truth!

---

## SECTION VI.

### *The conclusion.*

WHEN I consider the many seemingly plain and unequivocal marks of a good intention, and good disposition in Dr. Beattie, I am puzzled to account for his gross and injurious misrepresentations of the sentiments of his adversaries, and at the violence with which he is actuated, bordering sometimes upon a spirit of persecution.

'The

'The vulgar,' he ſays, p. 49, 'when 'they are puzzled with argument, have 'recourſe to their common ſenſe, and 'acquieſce in it ſo ſteadily, as often to 'render all the acts of the logician in- 'effectual; *I am confuted, but not con- 'vinced,* is an apology ſometimes offered 'when one has nothing to oppoſe to the 'arguments of the antagoniſt; but the 'original undiſguiſed feelings of his own 'mind. This apology is, indeed, very 'inconſiſtent with the dignity of philoſo- 'phic pride, which, taking for granted 'that nothing exceeds the limits of hu- 'man capacity, profeſſes to confute what- 'ever it cannot believe, and, which is ſtill 'more difficult, to believe whatever it 'cannot confute; but this apology may 'be perfectly conſiſtent with ſincerity and 'candour, and with that principle, of 'which Pope ſays, that, *though no ſcience, 'it is fairly worth the ſeven.*'

Now what is this but inſinuating, nay it is ſomething more than inſinuating, that all thoſe who do not admit this new doc- trine

trine of *the infallibility of common ſenſe*, are poſſeſſed of ſo much philoſophic pride, that they take it for granted that nothing can exceed the limits of their capacity; that we profeſs to confute whatever we cannot believe, and to believe whatever we cannot confute. But whatever effect this repreſentation may have upon thoſe who, knowing but little of men and books, are diſpoſed to take for granted whatever ſuch a man as Dr. Beattie will venture to aſſert ſo roundly, it is a mere chimera of his own brain: and this mode of writing is a moſt unjuſtifiable method of drawing an odium upon his opponents, who, perhaps, have no more philoſophic pride than himſelf. If arrogance and inſolence be an indication of pride, Dr. Beattie has certainly no ſmall ſhare of it, though it may hitherto have eſcaped his own ſearch.

His tacking the doctrine of neceſſity to the end of a liſt of peculiarly obnoxious and atheiſtical tenets, as if it was the natural and neceſſary completion of the whole ſcheme, in the preceding quota-

tion,

tion, is another inſtance of his unfairneſs, that looks very like *artifice;* and which I think exceedingly unjuſtifiable. A little of *irony* and *ſatyr*, and ſomething approaching to *aſperity*, may, perhaps, be indulged, as in a manner neceſſary to enliven controverſial writing; at leaſt it may be apologized for, as almoſt unavoidably ſuggeſted by the heat of debate; but the paſſages I have quoted above have a very different and a more malignant aſpect.

Dr. Beattie's vehemence, and his antipathy to thoſe who differ from him, though he is quite a *volunteer* in the controverſy, and cannot plead that he was heated by any *perſonal oppoſition*, approaches too near to the ſpirit of perſecution. At leaſt I do not ſee how elſe to interpret the following paſſage, and I earneſtly wiſh that the ingenuous author would do it himſelf, and help us, if it be poſſible, to interpret it without having recourſe to ſo unfavourable a comment. 'Had I,' p. 20, 'done 'but half as much as he (Mr. Hume) in

' labour-

'labouring to ſubvert principles which 'ought ever to be held ſacred, I know not 'whether the *friends of truth* would have 'granted me any indulgence, I am ſure 'they ought not. Let me be treated with 'the lenity due to a good citizen no longer 'than I act as becomes one.'

Certainly the obvious conſtruction of this paſſage is, that Mr. Hume ought not to be treated with the indulgence and lenity due to a good citizen, but ought to be puniſhed as a bad one. And what is this but what a Bonner or a Gardiner might have put into the preamble of an order for his execution. Judging, as Dr. Beattie does, by his own ideas of the tendency of principles, expreſſed in this book, he will, I doubt not, think ſeveral of my writings, if they have happened to fall in his way, and eſpecially theſe remarks on his treatiſe (in which I own I have endeavoured to lay the ax to the very root of his fundamental principles of virtue, religion and truth) to be equally dangerous, provided he ſhould think them in equal danger of ſpreading;

and,

and, if he be conſiſtent with himſelf, and think me worthy of his notice, I ſhall expect, after a ſummary proceſs before the tribunal of his common ſenſe, to be conſigned to the diſpoſal of his *friends of truth*, who may not be equally the friends and lovers of *mercy*. But, thanks to a good ſuperintending providence, which influences the hearts, and directs the affairs of men, our governors either do not entertain the ſentiments, or are not inſpired with the zeal of our author.

Dr. Beattie and I muſt certainly think and feel very differently with reſpect to many things. His dread of infidel writings, and his apprehenſion of the miſchief they may do, far exceeds mine. 'The 'writings of Mr. Hume,' he ſays, p. 472, 'notwithſtanding their obſcurity, have 'done miſchief enough to make every 'ſober-minded perſon earneſtly wiſh that 'they had never exiſted.'

Now I, for my part, am truly pleaſed with ſuch publications as thoſe of Mr. Hume,

Hume, and I do not think it requires any great ſagacity, or ſtrength of mind, to ſee that ſuch writings muſt be of great ſervice to religion, natural and revealed. They have actually occaſioned the ſubject to be more thoroughly canvaſſed, and conſequently to be better underſtood than ever it was before; and thus *vice cotis funguntur*.

In what a wretched ſtate would chriſtianity have univerſally been at preſent, loaded with ſuch abſurdities and impieties as all the eſtabliſhments of it contain, (that of Scotland by no means excepted) if it had not been for ſuch a ſcrutiny into it as the writings of unbelievers have promoted, and indeed have made abſolutely neceſſary.

Infidelity appears to me to have been the natural and neceſſary produce of corrupted chriſtianity; but I have no doubt but that this evil will find its own remedy, by purging our religion of all the abſurdities it contains, and thereby enabling it to triumph over all oppoſition. Things are now in ſuch a train that infidelity will have every day leſs and leſs to carp at in chriſtianity, till at length its excellence and divine authority will be univerſally acknowledged.

# REMARKS

ON

# Dr. OSWALD's APPEAL

TO

# COMMON SENSE

IN BEHALF OF

# RELIGION.

THE

# INTRODUCTION.

THE controverſy in which I am now engaged may perhaps illuſtrate the propriety of the old Latin proverb *Principiis obſta.* Dr. Reid's new principle of *Common ſenſe*, or, to give it a name leſs ambiguous, and more appropriated to its office, his *ſenſe of truth*, notwithſtanding the prodigious aſſurance with which it was uſhered into the world, and notwithſtanding the manifeſt inconſiſtency there is between it and the fundamental principles of Mr. Locke, concerning the human mind, was ſuffered to paſs without any particular notice. I ſuppoſe becauſe no particular *uſe* was made of it. It was conſidered as nothing more than a new-faſhioned theory of the human mind, eagerly adopted and cried up by ſome, who, in my opinion, were very ſuperficial judges of ſuch things; while thoſe who thought with me, that the whole ſyſtem was ill founded, did not, I ſuppoſe, think it worth their while to make any oppoſition to it; concluding that in due time the futility of it could not fail to be ſeen through, when it would fall into oblivion of itſelf.

Preſently, however, we find two writers, men of ſome note, Dr. Beattie and Dr. Oſwald, ſeeing that this new doctrine of a ſenſe of truth was received without any oppoſition, beginning to avail themſelves of it for the defence of religion, and of ſome peculiar tenets of their own, in the regular proof of which they had been embarraſſed. Dr. Beattie, indeed, with ſome degree of moderation and timidity, and not much in the detail of things; but Dr. Oſwald with great particularity, and with as much bigotry and violence, as if his principles had been the eſtabliſhed faith of all mankind in all ages, and not, as in truth they are, a thing of yeſterday.

Finding

Finding this new power of the human mind to be decisive and irresistible within its jurisdiction, and requiring no aid from reason, he immediately sets about enlarging its province (as the English government have lately done that of Quebec) throwing into it, without any regard to reason or conscience, every thing that he thought of value, and which he had found any difficulty in defending upon other principles.

By this means he has eased himself at once of the defence of all the first principles, or, as he calls them, *primary truths of religion;* such as the being, the unity, the moral perfections, and providence of God, and of a future state; of the evidences also of christianity, and even many of his favourite and least defensible doctrines in the christian system. And, moreover, on this new ground, as from a sanctuary, he pours the grossest abuse both upon all unbelievers, and those who have opposed them on the principles of reason only; treating them alike as fools or mad-

 men.

men. Dr. Oswald's treatise, however, as well as Dr. Beattie's, has many admirers, both north and south of the Tweed.

Finding things in this situation, I own I was willing to interpose my feeble endeavours to put a stop to this sudden torrent of nonsense and abuse that is pouring down upon us from the North, though at the evident *risk of my character*, as Dr. Oswald, vol. 2, p. 328, will tell me, and laying my account with meeting all that magisterial insolence, which he, and indeed the whole *triumvirate*, have boldly assumed with respect to others.

But if this task should not be undertaken by some person, I am afraid we shall find these new principles extending their authority farther than the precincts of metaphysics, morals, religion, christianity, and protestantism, to which they have been hitherto confined. Papists may begin to avail themselves of them for the support of all those doctrines and maxims for which the powers of reason had proved insufficient;

insufficient; and politicians also, possessing themselves of this advantage, may venture once more to thunder out upon us their exploded doctrines of passive obedience and non-resistance. For having now nothing to fear from the powers of *reason*, and being encouraged by the example of grave divines and metaphysicians, they may venture to assert their favourite maxims with the greatest confidence; appealing at once to this ultimate tribunal of common sense, and giving out their own mandates as the decisions of this new tribunal. For every man will think himself authorized to assume the office of interpreting its decrees, as this new power holds a separate office in every man's own breast. Indeed our author has left the politician but little to do with respect to this doctrine, having ranked *obedience to the magistrate* among the primary truths of nature. p. 247.

Considering the very late origin of this new empire of common sense, its conquests, it must be confessed, have been pretty

pretty rapid; and as it has ſubdued all the regions of metaphyſics, morals, and theology in the ſpace of ten years, it may be computed that, with this addition of ſtrength, it may, in ten years more, complete the reduction of all the ſeven ſciences; when the whole buſineſs of *thinking* will be in a manner over, and we ſhall have nothing to do but to *ſee* and *believe*.

Now, being no friend to implicit faith, becauſe, perhaps, it has been no friend to me, I am willing to oppoſe the farther encroachments of this bold invader, before it be quite too late. And having already made two campaigns in this juſt cauſe, as it appears to me, I am now preparing for a third, which I foreſee will be more difficult and hazardous than both the former. Nevertheleſs I will not deſpair; ſince, if I fail, I ſhall, at leaſt, be intitled to the epitaph of Phaeton, *Magnis tamen excidit auſis.*

But, dropping this figure, I really am much more at a loſs how to anſwer Dr. Oſwald, than either Dr. Reid, or Dr. Beattie, on account of the great incoherence of his work, and his remarkably looſe and declamatory way of writing; on which account his argument is ſo involved, that there is hardly any ſuch thing as coming at it; ſo that, though I have often ſaid, that if I have any talent, it is a facility in arrangement, I own that, for once, I have been exceedingly puzzled, and do not clearly ſee my way. I ſhall proceed, however, in the beſt manner that I can; giving, in the firſt place, the hiſtory of this new ſcience, as deduced by our author; then explaining the nature and extent of it; after which I ſhall ſhow more particularly the relation it bears to reaſoning, and point out ſome particular applications that our author has made of it.

In all this I ſhall do little more than ſelect and arrange a number of paſſages that I have collected from our author.

For

For I muſt acknowledge, that if he has embarraſſed me, and taken up my time in the diſpoſition of my materials, he has made me amends by ſaving me the trouble of making many obſervations. In fact, I ſhall have occaſion to do little more than let our author ſpeak for himſelf, only putting his words a little nearer together than he would have done. And as our author ſeems to have had great ſatisfaction in the firſt publication of his work, I hope he will not be diſpleaſed at this *new edition* of it. For whatever my reader may think of him as a *reaſoner*, my quotations cannot fail to verify the character that Dr. Beattie (whoſe judgment in this caſe no perſon will call in queſtion) gives of him, viz. that he is an *elegant writer*.

SEC-

## SECTION I.

### *Of the* Hiſtory *of Common ſenſe.*

IT has been a great loſs to hiſtory, that the principal actors in many great achievements have not themſelves written the hiſtory of them. But Dr. Oſwald has taken ſufficient care that there ſhould be no complaint of this kind with reſpect to the late triumph of *ſenſe* over *reaſon*. For though he himſelf is but the ſecond in ſucceſſion from Dr. Reid, who planned and began the attack, he has taken an opportunity of fully ſtating the ground of the war, and informing us of the progreſs that his predeceſſor had made in it.

The more fully to explain the riſe of this new ſyſtem, our author goes back to the times preceding the reformation from popery. Speaking of this popiſh darkneſs, he ſays, p. 52, 'Upon conſulting 'the ſacred records, and appealing to 'them' (not *reaſoning* from them) 'one

'half

'half of Chriſtendom were made ſenſible 'of their folly, and ſhook off the domi- 'nion of ignorance and error.——They 'ſplit again into ſects, formed different 'creeds, and different plans of worſhip 'and government; and having been 'much exerciſed in ſubtle and hot diſ- 'putes with the Romiſh doctors, they 'entered into conteſts of much the ſame 'kind, and in much the ſame ſpirit, with 'one another, about their peculiar tenets. 'Mean time, a ſect aroſe who called the 'whole in queſtion; and, believing them- 'ſelves equally privileged with others to 'ſound unfathomable depths, they em- 'ployed the ſame ſubtlety of reaſoning 'againſt religion which contending di- 'vines had employed againſt each other; 'and the friends of religion, not aware 'of the conſequence, did partly from 'their zeal for the truth, and partly from 'a habit of diſputing, and a confidence 'of victory, admit the whole to debate.'

Religion being now, through the fatal imprudence of its beſt friends, and the ableſt

ableſt that the times (which produced no ſuch men as Dr. Reid, Dr. Beattie, or Dr. Oſwald) afforded, become a ſubject of debate, divines were obliged to make the beſt of the arms with which they were furniſhed for the engagement. How things were conducted before the time of Mr. Locke our author does not particularly ſay; but though his writings were univerſally thought to be of great advantage to the cauſe of truth and religion, yet Dr. Oſwald informs us that he ſet out wrong, and thereby gave the enemy too great advantage.

'Mr. Locke, p. 108, unfortunately, 'derived all our knowledge from ſenſa'tion or reflection, intirely overlooking 'another principle, more important than 'them both, and without which they are 'of no avail. Senſation and reflection,' our author ſays, 'do indeed give occaſion 'to all our ideas, but they do not pro'duce them. They may, in our preſent 'ſtate, be conſidered as the *ſine qua non* 'to our moſt rational and ſublime con'ceptions,

'ceptions, but are not therefore the pow-'ers by which we form them. Thefe 'conceptions are formed in us by another 'and different power, which Mr. Locke, 'and unhappily, after him, the bulk of 'the learned, have overlooked. In this, 'p. 109, he has committed a capital over-'fight of very bad confequence. He has 'not only put the learned upon a falfe 'fcent, but has brought the primary 'truths of nature under fufpicion, and 'opened a door to univerfal fcepticifm.'

At this door, fet open by Mr. Locke, Mr. Hume and others have found admiffion. 'Hence, p. 110, difputes 'upon the moft important fubjects have 'been maintained, to the detriment of 'religion, and the difgrace of the human 'underftanding; nor will it be poffible 'to put an end to thefe difputes, without 'fearching farther into the powers of the 'human mind than Mr. Locke has done.'

To purfue this curious hiftory a little farther, 'Mr. Hume had penetration

'enough,'

'enough,' p. 110, 'to perceive the defect 'of Mr. Locke's hypothesis. but had not 'the courage to supply that defect, by the 'only way in which it could be supplied. 'Perhaps he suspected that philosophers 'would not submit to the authority of 'common sense, or was himself too much 'a philosopher to have recourse to an 'authority so vulgar and homely. He 'therefore found himself under a necessity of making the best account he 'could of the phenomena of nature by 'the received doctrine of the connection 'and association of ideas; and it must 'be owned that his account is extremely 'ingenious.'

'The author of the *Essays on the principles of morality and natural religion*, 'published Edinburgh, 1751,' p. 94, 112, 'alarmed at Mr. Hume's confounding 'rational belief with credulity, and denying the connection between cause and 'effect, has said all that is necessary in 'confutation of his opinion; but he has 'confuted Mr. Hume upon principles too

'much a-kin to his own. He has recouſe
'to our being ſo conſtituted that we muſt
'perceive, feel, and believe certain truths,
'without laying open the human conſti-
'tution, or once attempting to point out
'that in our frame which produces the
'way of thinking, which he juſtly ſays is
'unavoidable. That certain perſons are
'ſo conſtituted is perhaps all the account
'that can be made of odd and fanciful
'perceptions or feelings; but a more ſa-
'tisfactory account ought to be given of
'the primary truths of nature. He has
'not beſtowed that attention on the lead-
'ing power which is due; nor ſeems he
'to have reached a true and full view of
'the characteriſtic of a rational being.'
p. 114.

After theſe groſs blunders of Mr. Locke, Mr. Hume, and the author of the Eſſays, it is pleaſing to obſerve the approach that was made towards the diſcovery of this great principle of common ſenſe by Mr. Hutcheſon. 'Mr. Hutche-'ſon,' p. 158, 'thought that he had made

'a diſ-

'a diſcovery of a new faculty of the human mind, which he was intitled to call by a new name, and thereby gave offence to the friends of demonſtration; but in reality this great philoſopher had only got a view, and but a partial view of common ſenſe.'

Behold, however, at length, the great *deſideratum* completely diſcovered; and, after this ſtate of deplorable darkneſs and obſcure gueſſings, full day light is diffuſed by Dr. Reid. 'Dr. Reid,' vol. 2, p. 329, 'has put an effectual ſtop to the artifices of ſceptics, by pointing out three powers of the mind, evidently diſtinct, and eaſily diſtinguiſhed,' meaning perception, memory, and imagination; the operations of two of which imply the belief of the real exiſtence of their reſpective objects. 'We have found then,' ſays our author, p. 268, 'a ſource of ideas that has been too long overlooked, and in it have found the much conteſted ſource of moral obligation. Theology and ethics are now to be 'considered as a real ſcience, founded on 'principles of indubitable certainty; prin- 'ciples, which, if they are not as much 'regarded, are, however, intitled to equal 'regard with the axioms of the ſchools— 'the principles of *common ſenſe.*'

'Of late, p. 168, there has appeared '*An inquiry into the human mind, on the* '*principles of common ſenſe*, by Dr. Reid, 'in which he gives ſuch an account of the 'operations of our powers, as ſhews it to 'be impoſſible for a rational being to 'doubt the reality of the objects of ſenſe, 'and gives us ground to expect, from a 'farther purſuit of his inquiry, ſuch a diſ- 'play of the powers of the human mind, 'as will render it impoſſible for any one 'to doubt of the obvious truths of religion 'and virtue, without being convicted of 'folly or madneſs; ſo that the triumph of 'truth over error, and of true ſcience over 'falſe philoſophy may not be very diſtant.

'Upon the whole, p. 169, we are ar- 'rived at a period, in which, if it is not

'our

'our own fault, we may diſmiſs frivolous 'controverſies, and ſettle in the belief of 'primary truth upon the moſt ſolid foun-'dation.'

It is my *misfortune*, or, as Dr. Oſwald ſays above, my *fault*, that I cannot as yet diſmiſs all controverſy, and ſettle upon this ſolid foundation.

---

## SECTION II.

### *Of the* nature, limits, *and general* uſe *of the principle of Common ſenſe.*

HAVING ſeen the hiſtory of this great diſcovery deduced, with a ſolemnity worthy of its importance, my reader, if I had not in ſome meaſure gratified his curioſity already, in my account of Dr. Reid's and Dr. Beattie's performances, would have been impatient to be informed more particularly what this common ſenſe is. I can promiſe him, however, that though he has ſeen much, there is more to be ſeen; and that he will get new light and information from this and the following ſections.

In the firſt place, I ſhall preſent him with Dr. Oſwald's idea of the *nature, limits,* and *general uſes* of the faculty of common ſenſe.

According to our author, this new-diſcovered faculty is the 'leading and ſu-'preme power of the rational mind,' as he deſcribes it in the following paſſage, in which he alſo moſt pathetically laments that it has been hitherto much over-looked and neglected.

'The powers of compounding,' p. 86, 'dividing, and abſtracting our ideas have 'been unfolded with the greateſt accu-'racy and judgment; but its leading 'power, that which is ſupreme in the 'rational mind, and is its chief preroga-'tive and characteriſtic, has been much

'neg-

'neglected. Its objects are not enume-'rated, its extent is not known, and its 'authority is little regarded. For which 'reason a standard of theologic, ethic, 'and political truth is to this hour a *desi-'deratum* with the learned. On all these 'subjects we are become expert reason-'ers, but hardly know when or where to 'stop, or how to form a firm and steady 'judgment.'

The great importance of this principle may farther appear from the following censure of Mr. Locke. 'There is a ne-'cessity of declaring,' p. 70, 'in plain 'terms, that Mr. Locke, in his account 'of the origin of our ideas, is guilty of 'an oversight of very bad consequence. 'If, as our author represents, we can 'have no ideas besides those arising im-'mediately from impressions made on our 'organs of sense, or our own reflections 'upon those, then the authority of com-'mon sense must go for nothing, and a 'free scope is given to scepticism with re-

'spect to all truths that are not the im-
'mediate objects of sense.'

If we ask why this new faculty is to be called *sense*, or *common sense* (for as to a regular *definition*, that he absolutely declines giving us, leaving us to make it out as we can) he answers as follows, 'This characteristic power of the rational 'mind,' vol. 2, p. iv, *Advertisement*, 'on 'account of its quickness, clearness, and 'indubitable certainty, is called sense, and 'on account of its being possessed in one 'degree or other by all of the rational 'kind, is called common sense.' In this I would observe that our author differs from Dr. Beattie, who only says that this common sense is given to *a great majority of mankind*.

The great use of this common sense is that, instead of having *perceptions* or *emotions* for its object, like the other senses, it is employed about the more important business of *truth*, which it suggests without

out the help of any proper evidence; and yet it is the means of making the greateſt and moſt important diſcoveries.

'Mr. Locke unhappily overlooked the 'chief inlet to truth,' vol. 2, p. 42. 'That 'diſcoveries may be made in the arts and 'ſciences by reaſoning will not be denied; 'but that diſcoveries more numerous, 'more uſeful, and more certain may be 'made in both by a judicious attention 'to the operations of nature, cannot be 'doubted.' p. 34.

But the moſt important uſe of this new principle is derived from its relation to *morals*. It is 'the faculty of diſtin-'guiſhing between fit and unfit, right 'and wrong in conduct.' p. 119.

This principle of common ſenſe our author alſo conſiders as 'the *charac-'teriſtic of rationality*,' p. 102. 'We 'are not diſtinguiſhed, he ſays, p. 114, 'from ideots and the lower animals by 'perceptions, feelings, and inſtinctive

emo-

'emotions. We have perceptions ſpeci-'fically different from theſe, which the 'lower animals have not,' p. 116, 'viz. 'the perception of obvious truth and pal-'pable abſurdity,' p. 117. 'Mr. Locke,' p. 179, 'was guilty of a capital overſight, 'in making abſtraction the characteriſtic 'of rationality. There is another faculty 'which makes a yet more perfect diſtinction 'between men and brutes, the faculty, to 'wit, of perceiving and pronouncing upon 'the connection which ſubſiſts between 'qualities and powers, and the ſubjects to 'which they belong; of which faculty if 'the brutes were poſſeſſed, there ſeems no 'ground to doubt of their power of ab-'ſtracting, occaſionally, thoſe qualities 'and powers, in the ſame manner we do.'

So plain is it, that it is this common ſenſe that makes the difference between men and the lower animals, that, according to our author, none but thoſe who are themſelves ideots can doubt of it. 'That 'we are diſtinguiſhed by a ſet of ideas, 'and a ſyſtem of knowledge ſpecifically 'different

'different from theirs (the brutes) might 'without more ado be appealed to the 'breast of every man who is above the 'rank of an ideot; were it not that the 'learned lay us under a necessity of giv'ing them in detail.' p. 189.

It is the possession of this faculty of common sense that distinguishes men from *ideots* no less than from the lower animals. 'The characteristic of ideotism 'consists in an incapacity to distinguish 'between chance and design.' Vol. 2. p. 55.

We shall now consider how this new faculty is to be distinguished from the old ones, and first from *intuition;* with respect to which we shall find there has been some little fluctuation in our author's judgment, which appears to be rather unusual with him.

'The man who from the looks, ge'stures, and speech of his adversary, sees 'rage and resentment, which are not,

'strictly

'ſtrictly ſpeaking, objects of intuition, 'has the ſame information of thoſe paſ-'ſions as he has of any other reality, which 'he perceives intuitively by his external 'and internal ſenſes,' p. 238. 'If I be 'aſked whether primary truths are diſco-'vered by intuition, the anſwer will be in 'the negative; becauſe intuition has been 'confined to our perceptions of the ob-'vious relations and qualities of being.' But he affirms, at the ſame time, that our knowledge of primary truths is equally certain and indubitable as that of intuition. p. 238.

Afterwards our author owns that the knowledge we acquire by common ſenſe is properly intuitive. 'I was,' ſays he, p. 357, 'too ſcrupulous on that occaſion. 'Our knowledge of primary truth has an 'equal title with our knowledge of all 'other ſelf-evident truths to be reſolved 'into intuition.'

Our author diſtinguiſhes the informations of common ſenſe from thoſe of *ex-*

*perience,*

*perience*, as being more certain. 'I do 'not,' p. 361, 'found our belief of primary truths on experience alone; for 'experience alone doth not produce certainty.——The unthinking part of mankind,' p. 363, 'are often governed ſolely 'by experience, in much the ſame manner as children and ideots; but men of 'underſtanding ſearch for a more firm 'foundation of their faith.—The vulgar 'are not accurate reaſoners, and yet you 'will find that they do not chuſe to reſt 'in experience alone.'

It has been ſeen above that our author complains of the author of the Eſſays for confuting Mr. Hume upon principles too near a-kin to his own. However I muſt own that, for my part, I can ſee no material difference between the ſentiments of the author of the Eſſays, as explained by our author, and thoſe of Dr. Oſwald himſelf. 'He has recourſe,' ſays our author, p. 112, 'to our being ſo conſtituted that 'we muſt perceive, feel, and believe certain truths, without laying open the

'human

'human conſtitution, or once attempting 'to point out that in our frame which 'produces a way of thinking, which he 'juſtly ſays is unavoidable.' Now it appears to me that all the more ſatisfactory account that Dr. Oſwald himſelf can give of this part of our conſtitution, and all that he and Dr. Reid have done towards *laying it open*, is merely verbal, viz. giving a name to this unknown ſomething, calling it *common ſenſe*. But what addition is this to our knowledge of the ſubject?

Our author appears to be a little embarraſſed about the boundary between the province of *reaſon* and that of common ſenſe in the buſineſs of inferring the laws of nature from the phenomena. This has hitherto been aſcribed to reaſon, but our author, deſirous to find ſufficient employment for his new principle, is unwilling to admit of this, except in a qualified ſenſe. 'It is common to ſay,' p. 235, 'that we infer the laws of nature from 'the phenomena; but that way of ſpeak-

'ing

'ing is not philoſophically, nor ſtrictly 'true. In every juſt inference there is a 'reference to ſome well known truth, by 'the help of which the inference is made, 'and on the truth of which its juſtneſs 'depends. But there is no truth in na-'ture by which we can infer thoſe realities 'which are not the objects of ſenſe from 'thoſe that are. From the appearance 'of ſmoke we infer fire. Why? Becauſe 'we know the connection between the 'one and the other. Thus ſome general 'truth is always underſtood, on the 'knowledge of which the inference de-'pends.

But he afterwards ſays, 'If any,' vol. 2, p. 36, 'chuſe to ſay that they infer the 'primary truths from the phenomena, 'we allow the phraſeology, upon condi-'tion they keep in mind, that the inference 'reſults immediately and unavoidably 'from due attention to the object, and 'without the help of any middle term. 'Or if they chuſe to call ſuch obvious 'and neceſſary deductions reaſoning, we 'will

'will not diſpute about a word, provided 'they allow that ſuch reaſoning is not ſub'ject to the danger of thoſe errors and 'miſtakes we are liable to in every other 'exerciſe of the diſcurſive faculty.'

Some of the dictates of this general principle of common ſenſe, our author informs us, are the mathematical axioms; and the difference between theſe and other primary truths he explains as follows. 'The difference between the evidence 'for mathematical axioms and that which 'we have for other primary truths is 'merely circumſtantial,' p. 139. 'In 'judging of mathematical axioms you ſee 'the ground on which you proceed, 'which you do not ſee in judging of many 'other truths, on which we pronounce 'with equal certainty,' vol. 2, p. 324. So that whether we ſee the ground on which we walk, or not, we may proceed with equal confidence, being equally ſecure from falling.

## SECTION III.

*Of the* ſufficiency *and* univerſality *of the principle of Common ſenſe*

CONSIDERING the very important nature, high rank, and authority of common ſenſe, my reader will be pleaſed to be informed of the *ſufficiency* and *univerſality* of it, and of the confidence with which its dictates may, and ought to be delivered, whenever ſceptical reaſoners call them in queſtion.

'The principles of good ſenſe are ſo 'plain,' ſays our author, p. 17, 'that to 'illuſtrate and inculcate them is to tire 'the patience, and affront the judgment 'of the reader. The human mind,' p. 8, 'has a power of pronouncing, at firſt 'ſight, on obvious truth with a quickneſs, 'clearneſs, and indubitable certainty, ſi-'milar, if not equal, to the information 'conveyed by the external organs of 'ſenſe. Its exerciſe begins in children 'with the firſt dawn of rationality, and 'not till then; and is ever after enjoyed, 'in ſome degree, by learned and un- 'learned, and by every individual of the 'human kind, who is not an ideot, and 'ſomehow diſordered in his intellectuals. 'No man can be at a loſs,' p. 249, 'to 'know the propoſitions that are the ob- 'jects of common ſenſe from thoſe that 'are not, and to determine with himſelf 'whether he has, or has not, a right to 'ſuſpend his judgment.'

Conſidering that the dictates of this common ſenſe are ſo *clear*, and likewiſe *univerſal*, our author muſt not be cenſured when he treats thoſe who do not liſten to them with a ſeverity ſuited to their deſperate folly and madneſs; even though upon ſome particular occaſions he ſhould ſo far tranſgreſs the ſcripture rule, as to call his brother a *fool*.

'If your adverſary,' p. 12, 'have the 'boldneſs to queſtion the truth of firſt 'principles, or to ſubſtitute chimeras, 'inſtead

'instead of principles, you must necessarily appeal to common sense; and if you 'do so, you must show him how far he 'deviates from the standard appealed to, 'i. e. in other words you must convict 'him of *nonsense*. The harsh expression 'may, and ought to be avoided, but the 'idea conveyed by it must be kept in 'view. Without that you do nothing. 'Your appeal will be found frivolous 'and unjust.'

'It is impossible,' p. 134, 'to observe 'inferior animals move hither and thither 'by the direction of their appetites and 'inclinations without conceiving the idea 'of that self-determining power by which 'they act, &c. If any one has attended 'to such operations, without arriving at 'the knowledge and belief of such principles of action, we do not blame the 'dulness or slowness of his apprehension, 'but without scruple pronounce him a '*fool*.'

So abundantly ſufficient are the dictates of this common ſenſe, that in many caſes they even ſuperſede all other helps to truth. With reſpect to religion more eſpecially we are much better without them. They only embarraſs and perplex us.

'I ſhould not be very glad,' ſays our author, p. 353, 'to ſee a demonſtration 'of the being and perfections of God that 'would ſtand the ſevereſt trial: For a de-'monſtration equal to any in Euclid could 'add nothing to the belief that every ratio-'nal being has of it. You may reſt 'aſſured,' p. 354, 'that the beſt proof 'or demonſtration of theſe truths is that 'you cannot admit the ſuppoſition of the 'contrary, without your being conſcious 'of your playing the *fool* or the *madman*.' He recommends, p. 92, 'aſſerting in a 'high tone, that no demonſtration is of 'equal force with common ſenſe, and no 'confutation can ſerve the intereſt of truth 'ſo effectually, as a plain conviction of 'nonſenſe. And therefore,' ſays he, 'it

'was

'was the bufinefs of divines and philofo-
'phers to have recourfe to the fimple de-
'cifion of common fenfe, on fubjects fo
'plain and important. Too much can
'hardly be faid,' p. 171, 'to perfuade
'men to put lefs confidence in the faculty
'of reafoning, and more in the faculty of
'judgment than they commonly do.'

Such firm hold have the principles of common fenfe on the bulk of mankind, that no perfon who has any regard to his reputation will ever dare to call them in queftion; fo that we may be perfectly eafy in refting the caufe of religion upon this folid foundation. 'If one incline,' vol. 2, p. 328, 'to fet afide the authority of 'reafon' (as diftinguifhed from *reafoning*, p. 327) 'and deliver himfelf over to fancy, 'he may ufe what freedoms he will with 'primary truths, but not with fafety to 'his character. One muft either admit 'all obvious truths, or fall under the im- 'putation of folly and nonfenfe. This 'is learned nonfenfe,' p. 327, 'and fo are 'all the surmises that can be offered 'against indubitable truths.'

Considering how amply the dictates of common sense are guarded by their own evidence, and the sanction of all mankind, in so much that every man must be conscious that he is *playing the fool or the madman* who shall presume to gainsay them, that he cannot do it *with safety to his character*, that every man who hears him has a right to tell him to his face that he *talks nonsense*, and even need not scruple to call him a *fool*, it is rather wonderful that our author should want any other guard for his primary truths; and yet he, as well as Dr. Beattie, gives hints that the *aid of the magistrate*, and a little wholesome severity, might not be improper; provided that, contrary to his expectation, the above mentioned guards should prove not to be quite sufficient for so great and good a purpose. But, in fact, no people have been so ready to have recourse to persecution, as those who

who have pretended to infallibility. This was the caſe both with the infallible church of Rome, and the no leſs infallible Calvin. Countenanced by theſe great examples, the patrons of common ſenſe, which is as infallible as either of them can pretend to be, need not be aſhamed to do as they did.

'All poſſible encouragement,' ſays our author, vol. 2, p. 335, 'ought to be given 'to rational and juſt, and all manner of 'diſcouragement to fooliſh and nonſen-'ſical way of talking. No pleaſantry, no 'vivacity, no appearance of wit and hu-'mour, ought to atone for nonſenſe on 'any ſubject, eſpecially in thoſe of the 'greateſt weight and importance. It 'were even to be wiſhed that the civil 'magiſtrate were authorized to put a 'ſtigma on palpable abſurdity, in ſub-'jects where the honour of God and the 'intereſt of mankind are deeply con-'cerned. But as this might be danger-'ous, it is alſo unneceſſary.'

## SECTION IV.

### *Of the natural* imperfections *and necessary* culture *of Common sense.*

LEST the idea which my reader will naturally conceive of the power and influence of common sense, from the contents of the last section, should lead him to expect from it more than he will find, it is necessary, before we proceed any farther, to apprize him, that here, as in many other cases (examples of which he will find in abundance in the prosecution of his studies) *fact* and *experience* do not exactly tally with the preconceived *theory*.

He would too naturally imagine that the principle which distinguishes *every individual of the human race*, being the very *characteristic of rationality*, which pronounces with *quickness*, *clearness*, and *indubitable certainty*, on *all primary truths*, and which was intended by our maker

maker to be an almoſt *infallible direction in the whole conduct of life*, and eſpecially in matters of *religion*, would be a ſovereign and effectual antidote, or rather preventive, of all error, impoſition and vice; and that upon this foundation the empire of truth and virtue would be ſecurely and for ever eſtabliſhed.

But, alas! our author, having, no doubt for good reaſons, given this exerciſe to our *imaginations*, thinks proper to give us a leſſon of humility, patience, and induſtry, by acquainting us, that, in fact, the dictates of common ſenſe are very little known or regarded in the world; for that, what through the leſſer encroachment of *vulgar prejudice* on one ſide, and the greater and bolder encroachments of *philoſophy* on the other, her authority is almoſt annihilated; ſo that almoſt all received opinions and eſtabliſhed maxims are fundamentally wrong.

All this, however, is eaſily explained and accounted for, by a little variation in the idea he had firſt given us of this wonderful power; and which, in fact, only ſerves to raiſe our admiration of it higher than ever. Before he compared it to a *ſenſe* in general, now it reſembles the moſt perfect of all the ſenſes the *eye*, which we have a power of rendering quite uſeleſs to us by covering it with the eye-lid, which nature has, to be ſure, provided for that purpoſe, leſt by the too free uſe both of the external and internal eye, we ſhould injure them, and thereby intirely deprive ourſelves of them. And though no man ever voluntarily ſhut up his external eyes, except to relieve them, and make them more ſerviceable to him afterwards; yet men are almoſt univerſally diſpoſed to do this with reſpect to the eye of the mind, taking particular pleaſure in the diverſion which in the country is called *blind-man's-buff*.

'As

'As the eye,' ſays our author, p. 361, 'has a power of letting in more or leſs 'light, ſo the mind has a power of ad'mitting theſe truths in a greater or leſs 'degree at pleaſure.'

Again, whereas the other ſenſes are improved by exerciſe to a certain degree, this internal ſenſe is capable of indefinite improvement, even *ad infinitum;* ſo that though the eye and ear admit of no ſenſible improvement from ten to fourſcore years, this *eye of the mind* is improved, as our author has found by computation, in an exact arithmetical ratio with the application of it. For with the eye of the mind you ſee every thing juſt a thouſand times better for having looked at them a thouſand times. A man, therefore, who has but juſt begun to make uſe of his common ſenſe is no more fit to hold an argument with a man who has grown expert in the uſe of it, than a man with his naked eyes only can diſpute about the ſpots of the ſun with one who has got a teleſcope. The latter ſees a thouſand

thouſand things in objects that the former cannot poſſibly ſee at all. How this can be reconciled with the fact, of mankind not improving in knowledge, but ſometimes going backwards, I leave to our author's *third* publication on the ſubject.

'It may ſeem a paradox,' ſays our author, vol. 2, p. 349, 'but it is a certain 'truth, that common ſenſe, as it is in'deed more worthy, ſo it is not leſs capa'ble of culture than any other of our fa'culties. We do not pretend,' p. 255, 'to determine the degree of certainty at 'which he will arrive, for that will be 'proportioned to the degree of rationa'lity of which he is poſſeſſed; but he 'may promiſe himſelf ſatisfaction ſuited 'to the exerciſe he gives his good ſenſe 'and probity on this important occaſion. 'This preſcription is no leſs proper for 'the unthinking part of mankind, than 'for profeſſed ſceptics. Many take pri'mary truths for granted, without at'tending to their evidence; who, if they 'took the trouble of comparing them 'with

'with the oppoſite abſurdities, would be-
'lieve them more cordially, and feel their
'influence upon the temper and manner
'more ſenſibly than they do.'

'He who has diſtinguiſhed fifty times,' vol. 2, p. 346, 'between obvious truth 'and arbitrary conceit, pronounces with 'a clearneſs of perſuaſion fifty times 'greater than that with which another 'pronounces, who has diſcerned the dif-'ference but once only; and he who has 'diſtinguiſhed a hundred times, pro-'nounces with a quickneſs and firmneſs 'a hundred times greater,' &c.

To improve upon this hint, ſuppoſe our author were to draw up a liſt of primary truths, get it printed, and, in order to employ the civil magiſtrate in *preventing* rather than *puniſhing* error, let him compel every child, from the very firſt dawn of rationality, to repeat them fifty or a hundred times every morning. We knew before that ſuch an exerciſe would ſtrengthen the *voice*, and now we have reaſon to think it would contribute no leſs to ſtrengthen the *judgment*. The danger would be leſt, by this exerciſe, mankind ſhould be too knowing for their rank in the creation.

This doctrine of Dr. Oſwald's, concerning the improveableneſs of the faculty of common ſenſe by culture, it may be proper to obſerve, is the very reverſe of Dr. Beattie's ſentiments on the ſame ſubject. In his compariſon of reaſon and common ſenſe, p. 47, he ſays, that the former is *more in our power* than the latter. He adds, 'There are few faculties, either of our mind or body, more improveable by culture than that of reaſoning; whereas common ſenſe, like other inſtincts, arrives at maturity with almoſt no care of ours.' This, and other points of difference, I hope theſe learned doctors will ſettle between themſelves, before they join their forces for their common defence.

This

This opening of the intellectual eye muſt, however, be a very diſagreeable and painful operation; or, ſince the advantages of keeping it open are ſo very great, one would think that men would have hit upon ſome contrivance to keep them always open. Whereas, on the contrary, they ſeem to have got ſome extraordinary, and moſt effectual method of keeping their eye-lids down.

'It is,' ſays our author, ſpeaking of common ſenſe, p. 17, 'the gift of heaven, 'but needs to be ſtirred up; and has been 'ſo long and univerſally neglected, that 'to give it full exerciſe, requires more 'attention, and application of thought, 'than moſt people are willing to beſtow. 'The principles of good ſenſe, ibid. are 'diametrically oppoſite to received opi-'nions, and eſtabliſhed maxims.'

But, notwithſtanding this, common ſenſe has more hold of the vulgar, than it has of the learned. 'There are thoſe,' p. 274, 'not indeed of the unlearned,

'but

'but among the learned, who diſtruſt the 'authority of common ſenſe, and ſeem 'to doubt its exiſtence; and ſome there 'are who poſitively affirm that there nei-'ther is, nor can be, any ſuch thing. In 'truth, the unlearned are the only peo-'ple who retain a clear idea of common 'ſenſe, and appeal to it as an oracle, and 'the learned only are ſceptical. You 'ſhall not find a man of ſenſe among the 'unlearned who heſitates, and ſcarce will 'you find one among the learned who 'doth not. Such are the bleſſed effects of 'modern learning.'

If the too ſagacious reader ſhould diſcover any thing like inconſiſtency between this quotation and the preceding, he ſhould conſider that, though I have brought them together, one of them is taken from p. 17, and the other from p. 274, which are ſufficiently diſtant from one another. In the following paragraphs our author explains the reaſon of this departure from common ſenſe, both in the vulgar and in the learned.

'As

'As the vulgar, through the groſſneſs 'of their conceptions, have lame and 'confuſed ideas of primary truths, ſo 'the learned have puzzled themſelves 'and others about them by the arts of 'reaſoning, to which they have been ſo 'long and ſo violently attached. So 'that, in fact, the common people de-'prive themſelves of the bleſſings of 'common ſenſe by thinking too little, 'and the learned by thinking too much.'

Beſides the general defects, and neglects, relating to this power of common ſenſe, it ſeems to be more eſpecially defective in its information concerning the *ſelf determining power*, which our author is reſolved to preſerve, though all mankind, at leaſt both the learned and unlearned, which I ſuppoſe includes them all, think differently from him on the ſubject. 'Notwithſtanding our averſion 'to frivolous diſputes,' vol. 2, p. 208, 'about obvious truths, ſomething muſt 'be done to give ſatisfaction concerning 'a ſelf determining power. Otherwiſe 'all that has been ſaid, or can be ſaid, in 'favour of virtue, muſt go for nothing; 'becauſe all men, learned and unlearned, 'bigots or free-thinkers, are not merely 'ſceptical, but infidels with regard to the 'reality of this power.' It is, indeed, very ſtrange, but not the leſs true, that all mankind ſhould be poſſeſſed of this moſt important power, on which all virtue depends, and yet that they ſhould be ſo far from knowing, or ſuſpecting it, and that they cannot be perſuaded to believe they have any ſuch thing. This ſomething reſembles Moliere's *Medecin malgrè lui.*

## SECTION V.

*Of the extenſive application of the principle of common ſenſe to* morals *and* religion.

THIS life is nothing but a ſcene of joys and ſorrows, hopes and fears; and we are continually paſſing from the one to the other. All this will be frequently exemplified by my reader. And as I firſt gave him a general view of the bright ſide of my picture, and then deſired him to contemplate the ſhade, I ſhall now exhibit the bright ſide again, and deſire him to take a more particular ſurvey of it.

We ſhall here find that this great oracle of the human breaſt has pronounced moſt diſtinctly concerning all the fundamental doctrines and duties of morality, comprehending the whole of natural religion, the evidences of chriſtianity, and even the more eſſential articles of chriſtian faith. To this, however, we muſt ſubjoin our author's juſt, pathetic, and eloquent complaints of the ſhameful neglect of this principle; and the great folly of philoſophers and divines in having recourſe to the deceitful principle of *reaſon;* which, according to our author, may almoſt be conſidered as the ſource of all evil and miſchief; when every thing they ought to have wiſhed for might have been obtained without any trouble at all, by only applying to common ſenſe.

Speaking of the great outlines of morality in general, our author ſays, vol. 2, p. 195, 'The obligations ariſing from 'obvious relations are the objects of 'common ſenſe.' Again, p. 24, 'Beſides 'thoſe inſtinctive emotions and feelings, 'which we have in common with the 'lower animals, every individual of the 'human kind has a perception, which 'ideots and the inferior animals have 'not, of what he owes to himſelf, to his 'offspring, to his friends, and benefac'tors, to his country, and to his God.— 'Thoſe ſacred obligations, which have 'been

'been the ſubject of diſpute with the 'learned, are objects of ſimple per-'ception and judgment to men of ſenſe.'

'That magiſtrates ought to be obeyed,' p. 247, 'that the workman is worthy of 'his wages, that every one ought to take 'care of his own, and his family's intereſt, 'and that men ought to do kind and 'friendly offices to each other; theſe, 'and the like propoſitions, appear obvi-'ouſly true, as the propoſitions oppoſite 'to them appear obviouſly falſe, to every 'man of common ſenſe.'

Such are the dictates of our infallible inſtructor and guide as to the great duties of morality, reſpecting this life. If we want to be informed concerning the peculiar *ſanctions* of natural religion, our author aſſures us, p. 8, that this great principle 'affords men an almoſt infal-'lible direction in the whole conduct of 'their lives, and that it was intended by 'the author of our being for giving us 'intire ſatisfaction concerning all primary

 'truths,

'truths, thoſe of religion in particular; 'and that our not having recourſe to this 'power is the true cauſe of thoſe idle diſ'putes, which have been maintained of 'late about the truth of religion.'

That the *being* of God ought not to be attempted to be proved by reaſon we have in ſome meaſure ſeen already, and we ſhall hear more on that ſubject hereafter; we ſhall, therefore, proceed to other articles of religion. 'To acknowledge the being, 'and diſpute the *attributes* of God, be'trays,' ſays our author, vol, 2, p. 80, 'great ſtupidity, or groſs prevarication.' Now for the divine *unity*. 'A work of de'ſign,' vol. 2, p. 75, 'indicates one and 'but one author to a ſound underſtand'ing.' With reſpect to the obligation to *worſhip* and *obey* God, he acknowledges, indeed, p. 216, that 'it would be un'reaſonable to expect the ſame inſtinctive 'emotions and inclinations that we have 'to the other offices of life. But,' he ſays, 'we have a clear perception of 'thoſe obligations, accompanied with

'emotions

'emotions and inclinations which nearly
'resemble those we call instinctive.'

Speaking of trusting in God, with respect to things that are above our comprehension, our author says, with peculiar emphasis and eloquence, vol. 2, p. 140, 'This is religion, this is philosophy, this 'is common sense. It is *nonsense*,' says he, vol. 2, p. 97, 'to talk of difficulties 'and embarrassments arising from a con'stitution of things to which the supreme 'being gave existence of his free choice.' Other divines are content with saying that this conduct is highly *unreasonable*.

The great difficulty in the theory of natural religion is the proof of a *future life*; but, happily, that difficulty is now intirely removed. Let us only silence the impertinence of reason, and common sense will speak plain enough, and to the purpose on this subject. 'We do not 'pretend,' says Dr. Oswald, vol. 2, p. 296, 'to demonstrate, from any thing that we know of the present state, that 'there will be a future ſtate of exiſtence.' This has been ſaid by many chriſtian divines, but then they have recourſe to revelation for a ſure foundation of their faith in this great doctrine; but our author can do without this reſource.

'We muſt,' ſays he, vol. 2, p. 306, 'enter a complaint againſt the learned of 'both ſides, for their injurious manner 'of treating this intereſting and impor- 'tant ſubject. In place of ſetting full in 'the view of mankind, a truth which 'none pretend to doubt of, and about 'which no man can be unconcerned, viz. 'that we are *accountable* to God for our 'conduct, the friends of religion and 'virtue have ranſacked all nature for 'arguments to prove that we ſhall *actu- 'ally be called to account*, and have there- 'by turned the attention of mankind 'from their proper buſineſs to an endleſs 'and fruitleſs diſpute, about what is poſ- 'ſible and impoſſible in nature, and may 'or may not come to paſs. Was this 'well adviſed? If a man is deſirous of 'certain

'certain information concerning this 'great event, let him consult the revelation which God has made of his mind. 'Or if he is not satisfied about that, let 'him consult the sentiments of his own 'heart, about his being *liable to account*. '——But if he will do neither, your reasoning is vain; for the man is a fool, 'and his folly is voluntary, and therefore incurable, or not to be cured by 'the art of reasoning.'

If my reader will not peruse this paragraph over again, he will perhaps overlook the most excellent *distinction without a difference*, with which the whole compass of his reading will ever furnish him. That we are *accountable to God* for our conduct, is a truth that no man can pretend to doubt of, or be unconcerned about; and yet all the powers of reason cannot persuade the same man to believe that he shall be *actually called to account*. And all the mischief that has been done by philosophers and divines has arisen from their not having attended to the diſtinction between thoſe two very different things.

Since this diſtinction is of ſuch unſpeakable conſequence, and has hitherto been intirely overlooked by all divines and philoſophers, it would certainly very much oblige and benefit the world if Dr. Oſwald would give us a diſcourſe upon the ſubject; inſiſting largely and ſtrongly on the conſideration of our being *accountable to God*, and being *liable to be called to account*, but, at the ſame time, carefully avoiding every thing that could give us an idea of our ever being *actually* brought to account. I the leſs wonder at the conduct of divines in this caſe, becauſe I think it muſt require no ſmall ingenuity and ſkill to do it. But what may not be expected from the eloquence of Dr. Oſwald!

Speaking more particularly of Socrates's arguments for a future ſtate, he ſays, vol. 2, p. 288, 'But in that variety 'of arguments, advanced by this great 'and

'and good man, none give ſuch ſatiſ-'faction to a plain underſtanding, as his 'obſervation to Crito, that the carcaſs he 'ſhewed ſo great concern about was not 'Socrates; that Socrates was he who 'then diſcourſed, reaſoned, and gave 'arrangements to his thoughts, and who, 'he ſaid, would ſoon give them the ſlip. 'This is common ſenſe.

Deriving ſo much information from common ſenſe, and finding ſuch effectual ſanctions of virtue in it, one would have thought that *revelation* might have been ſpared; and many good chriſtians would be exceedingly offended at our author for aſcribing ſo much to *nature* in this reſpect. But then he makes atonement, by eſtabliſhing the evidences of revelation upon the foundation of the ſame common ſenſe; which, of courſe, ſuperſedes all *reaſoning* about the matter, and thereby ſaves thoſe good chriſtians a great deal of trouble, in inquiring for themſelves, or replying to the impertinent cavils of others.

'Of

'Of a revelation from God,' meaning no doubt the Jewiſh and chriſtian, he ſays, p. 56, that 'few have any ſerious 'doubt, and that no man can diſbelieve 'it in any conſiſtency with common ſenſe.' But for the farther illuſtration of this important ſubject another whole volume is promiſed us.

As the truth of the ſcripture hiſtory is founded on common ſenſe, ſo we may take it for granted that its contents are agreeable to it. 'The ſcriptures,' ſays our author, vol. 2, p. 203, 'are the true, 'if not the only ſource of ſound philoſo-'phy and good ſenſe on theſe ſubjects, 'viz. moral obligation.' By the way, after making good ſenſe the ſource of ſo much knowledge in morals, I do not ſee with what propriety our author can call the ſcriptures the ſource of this good ſenſe.

The manner in which Dr. Oſwald ſpeaks of 'two important truths,' which, he ſays, the chriſtian revelation ſuperadds to our natural notions of religion, which it has revived,

revived, viz. 'an œconomy of grace in 'this life, and an exact retribution in the 'next,' is particularly curious. 'One 'cannot conceive,' says he, p. 254, 'what 'prejudice a man of sense can have to 'this plain doctrine. And as it was re-'ceived by persons no wise prejudiced in 'its favour, upon an attestation in which 'they could not be deceived, one must 'reckon all scepticism concerning it as 'mere affectation.' When a man speaks of indubitable truths he ought at least to use intelligible language; but what our author means by *an œconomy of grace*, I really do not understand.

I now come to present my reader with a few specimens of our author's pathetic and eloquent complaints on the subject of neglecting this common sense, in the defence of religion, natural and revealed, and on divines having imprudently condescended to reason about it, which was a piece of complaisance as mischievous as it was unnecessary. Infidels are a set of people with whom it is exceedingly improper

improper for a christian philosopher, and much beneath his dignity, to hold any parley.

'Is there not,' says Dr. Oswald, p. 364, 'just cause of complaint against the 'learned for overlooking distinctions 'which seldom escape the observation of 'the vulgar, and thereby exposing religion to objections which would be rejected with disdain on any other subject? 'Not only the christian revelation,' p. 55, 'but the moral perfections and government of God, yea and the very being 'of virtue, have been made the subject 'of dispute. Free-thinkers are not 'ashamed to publish their doubts concerning these realities, divines and philosophers have not disdained to establish 'them by a multitude of arguments.'

'The power of custom,' vol. 2, p. 152, 'in reconciling the mind to measures however absurd, which are become familiar, 'is almost incredible. Should an Indian 'of good sense be told, that for some 'time

'time paſt, men of the greateſt eminence 'in the learned world had been employed 'in diſputing with one another about the 'reality of virtue and vice; whether, 'for inſtance, the obligations of juſtice, 'temperance, gratitude, were nominal, 'fictitious and fanciful; or whether we 'were, indeed, bound to the practice of 'theſe and ſuch like virtues; that volumes 'have been written on both ſides, and 'deep attention given to the controverſy, 'and that each hypotheſis had its vo- 'taries; would the foreigner give credit 'to this report?

'Yet this conduct, ſo unaccountable 'to a foreigner, has been continued 'among us without much notice. The 'ſubject, it is true, merits the ſtricteſt 'attention; the reſearches on both ſides 'were curious enough, acquiſitions of 'ſome value were made in the abſtract 'ſciences; the audacity of one ſide ſeemed 'to require a check and the zeal of the 'other was at leaſt pardonable. But, in 'good earneſt, might not that zeal, that

'acute-

'acuteneſs, penetration, and compaſs of 'thought, have been employed with 'greater propriety, and to more advan-'tage? Was there any occaſion at all 'for ſuch diſquiſitions? Muſt metaphyſi-'cians and ſubtle diſputants be called in 'to evince our obligations to do the 'right and ſhun the the wrong? Can we, 'without renouncing common ſenſe, be 'ignorant, doubtful, or even inſenſible to 'ſuch obligations? There is need, great 'need, to awaken, revive, and enforce 'them; but without the influence of 'falſe learning there could be no room 'to doubt what every man of common 'underſtanding does, and muſt perceive 'at firſt ſight.'

How fatal would a ſtrict regard to *truth* be to a turn for *eloquence*. All this truly fine piece of declamation would have been loſt to the world, if our author had recollected, that *moral obligation itſelf* never was a ſubject of diſpute, but only the *foundation* of this obligation. Let our author endeavour to recollect the

the names of the writers who ever diſputed whether men were indeed bound to the practice of juſtice, temperance, &c.

Theſe complaints reſpect *writers* chiefly, but his complaints againſt the *preachers of the goſpel*, on the ſame ſcore, are ſtill ſtronger. 'What is more to be regretted,' ſays Dr. Oſwald, p. 56, 'the preachers 'of the goſpel, forgetting the dignity of 'their character, and the deſign of their 'office, have condeſcended to plead the 'cauſe of religion in much the ſame man-'ner as lawyers maintain a diſputed right 'of property. Inſtead of awakening the 'natural ſentiments of the human heart, 'and giving them a true direction, they 'have entered into reaſonings about 'piety, juſtice, and benevolence, too 'profound to be fathomed by the multi-'tude, and too ſubtle to produce any 'conſiderable effect. Inſtead of ſetting 'forth the diſplays of the divine perfec-'tions in the diſpenſation of the goſpel, 'ſo admirably fitted to touch, to pene-'trate, and to ſubdue the human mind, 'they have entertained their audiences 'with long and laboured proofs of a reve- 'lation from God, of which few have any 'serious doubt, and which no man can 'disbelieve in any consistency with com- 'mon sense. May not this be called, 'with propriety, a throwing cold water 'on religion? and ought it not to be 'considered as one of the chief causes of 'that insensibility to all its concerns of 'which we so frequently complain? The 'multitude has been astonished, wise men 'have been ashamed, and good men 'grieved at this treatment of religion, so 'much beneath its dignity.'

Our author intimates, however, that, bad as the case is, it is not yet quite desperate. Access to the tree of life is yet open, and common sense, this remedy for all our ills, though hitherto so shamefully neglected, will not refuse her succour upon proper application.

'Till divines and philosophers,' vol. 2, p. 221, 'have abated their ardour for fri-

'volous

'volous inquiries, and learned the art of 'turning the attention of mankind to ob-'vious and interesting truth, they have 'no title to complain of the unthinking 'part of mankind. For one may be bold 'to affirm, that multitudes would act a 'better part than they do, if they were 'under better treatment.' Now as Dr. Oswald's parish is undoubtedly under this very treatment, I should be glad to be informed of the state of it. Though his books have, in some measure, put all the world under the same treatment, it is too large a field of inquiry; and though I have read his performance with some degree of attention, there may be something in my particular constitution that *turns medicine into poison*. See p. 372.

'It is apparent,' says our author, vol. 2, p. 204, 'that if common sense had been 'consulted, a controversy of the most 'pernicious kind might have been wholly 'prevented, or soon stopped. And, if 'men will yet pay the regard that is 'due to common sense, they shall find 'themſelves relieved from embarraſſments 'they have always complained of, and 'ſee the whole of religion riſe to their 'view in that obvious, plain, and plea- 'ſant light, in which the face of nature 'appears when freed from thoſe miſts and 'clouds by which it was obſcured.'

Laſtly, our author proceeds to give more particular directions concerning what is neceſſary to be done by divines towards the reformation of the world, without addreſſing the reaſon of their hearers; which is a thing that they ought, if poſſible, to have nothing to do with. This is to put them under the direction of God, in the dictates of common ſenſe, when I put all the paſſages together, if I underſtand him rightly. For there is ſomething of the air of *myſticiſm* in what he ſays upon this ſubject; and things of that nature do not find the readieſt admiſſion to my underſtanding.

'Till divines and philoſophers,' vol. 2, p. 227, 'are better ſkilled in touching 'the

'the ſprings of the human heart than 'they are, or affect to appear, they can'not reach the end they propoſe; and 'were they poſſeſſed of all the eloquence 'of Greece or Rome, they could not ac'compliſh what they ought to have in 'view, I mean to ſave thoſe from ruin 'who will not take the trouble of ſaving 'themſelves; and in order thereto, to 'correct and cure the inveterate folly of 'the human heart. There is ſomething 'here that demands a deeper attention 'than has been given to it; ſomething too 'that points at a method of forming 'mankind to virtue which has been too 'much neglected.'

'The great ſecret informing men to 'religion and virtue,' vol. 2, p. 232, 'if 'it is fit to call that a ſecret which is ſo 'palpable to common ſenſe, and ought 'to have been publiſhed to all the world, 'is to perſuade them to reſign themſelves 'to God, as docile and dutiful pupils, to 'a faithful and capable tutor. To put 'mankind under a divine direction and 'influence,' vol 2, p. 229, 'ought to be 'the chief aim of all our inſtructors in 'religion and virtue. For without doing 'ſo, all their other preſcriptions will be 'found ineffectual, and indeed a mere 'project. All partial proceedings ought 'to be diſmiſſed, and juſtice done to pri- 'mary truths.' Vol. 2, p. 230.

---

## SECTION VI.

### *Of the incroachments of common ſenſe on the province of* Reaſon.

LEST Dr. Oſwald ſhould blame me for exhibiting his ſentiments without any proper refutation, which I have not always done, becauſe I really thought it to be needleſs, eſpecially after what I have ſaid in anſwer to his ſuperiors, Dr. Reid and Dr. Beattie; and alſo becauſe I thought it would be doing for my reader what he would very eaſily do for himſelf,

himſelf, and might rather chuſe to do for himſelf; I promiſe to be a little more ſerious in this and the following ſections; in the firſt of which I ſhall endeavour to ſhow that, as great an enemy as Dr. Oſwald is to reaſoning on the ſubject of morals and religion, he himſelf makes more uſe of it than he is willing to acknowledge. For, to make the more of his principle of common ſenſe, he has manifeſtly encroached upon what has hitherto been univerſally deemed the province of reaſon.

To prevent all miſtake of my meaning I ſhall here obſerve, that a propoſition may be ſaid to be proved by reaſon when a *third term* is neceſſary to ſhow the connection between the *ſubject* and *predicate* of it; and that a general propoſition is proved by an induction of a ſufficient number of the particulars which are comprized in it.

Thus, when I want to prove that the three internal angles of a right lined triangle are equal to two right angles, I make another ſet of angles, to which I know that the three angles in queſtion are equal, and which I can alſo eaſily ſhew to be equal to two right angles. If I want to prove that any particular perſon is generous, I point out a number of generous things that he has done, which indicate that character.

If our author will ſay that this is not reaſoning, I anſwer that then there is no ſuch thing as reaſoning. This, I will venture to ſay, has hitherto been univerſally deemed reaſoning; and if Dr. Oſwald chuſes to call it by any other name, he impoſes upon himſelf and the world, by changing the eſtabliſhed ſignification of words. But, in fact, it will appear, from a paſſage that I ſhall preſently quote, that Dr. Oſwald has the ſame ideas of the nature of reaſoning, though he ſeems very often to have loſt ſight of them.

That Dr. Oſwald, in many caſes, merely cavils at the terms *reaſon*, *proof*, and *demonſtration*, and that he miſapplies them, in order to ridicule and explode them, is very evident to me; and I think it cannot but appear ſo to all my readers, who are not quite adepts in this new ſcience of common ſenſe, and conſequently accuſtomed to the phraſes and ſenſe of terms peculiar to it.

Speaking of the being and attributes of God, he ſays, p. 151, 'To what purpoſe 'demonſtrate a truth, to the indubitable 'certainty of which all nature bears teſti-'mony.' Now excepting Dr. Clark's arguments *a priori*, which have long ceaſed to be ſo much as mentioned by divines, all that, in fact, has ever been meant by *demonſtrating* the being and attributes of God, is to exhibit and explain the teſtimony of nature; by pointing out ſuch marks of deſign, power, and benevolence in the conſtitution of the world, as prove not only that it had a cauſe, but that this cauſe muſt be a being

poſſeſſed

poſſeſſed of great power, wiſdom, and goodneſs.

Again he ſays, p. 197, 'You cannot 'form an idea of God, by gazing upon 'his works, without obſerving their ten-'dency; and entering as far as your 'faculties will carry you into his great, 'wiſe, and gracious plan.'

After our author has evinced the *being* of a God, without the help of reaſon, he proceeds to aſſert, in the title of the firſt chapter of book third, that 'to acknow-'ledge the being and diſpute the attri-'butes of God, betrays great ſtupidity, 'or groſs prevarication.' But the manner in which he ſupports this with reſpect to the particular attributes, is ſo like reaſoning, that I own I can ſee no difference between it and reaſoning. Let the reader judge.

'We acknowledge,' vol. 2, p. 81, 'that 'it is impoſſible to avoid the idea of God 'when we look on the phenomena of na-

'ture;

'ture; but if we do not content ourſelves 'with words without meaning, we muſt, 'at the ſame time, acknowledge, that it 'is impoſſible for us to form any concep-'tion of the immenſe ſyſtem of nature, 'without an idea of the immenſity of his 'power who made and upholds it; that 'it is impoſſible to trace the endleſs con-'nection and combination of cauſes con-'ſpiring to one great deſign, without 'having an idea of the unfathomable 'depth of the divine wiſdom; that it is 'impoſſible to ſurvey the multitude of 'living creatures he has brought into be-'ing, which he upholds in being, and 'protects from danger, and for whom he 'makes continual and bountiful ſupplies, 'without acknowledging his immenſe be-'nevolence and parental care. And 'when we recollect the various ſufferings 'of body and mind, which he has con-'nected with, and made conſequent upon 'almoſt every deviation from moral rec-'titude, even in this life, and the natural 'dread which every guilty perſon has of 'a more exact retribution in another ſtate,

'it

'it is impoſſible for us to avoid an idea 'of his tremendous juſtice.'

That any perſon ſhould be able to write this, and call it by any other name than *reaſoning* I own ſurprizes me not a little; and I can only compare our author to the poor man who had ſpoken *proſe* all his life without knowing it.

Alſo when Dr. Oſwald ſays, p. 138; 'It is *nonſenſe* to expect that lead ſhould 'ſwim in water,' it is impoſſible that his meaning ſhould really differ from that of the generality of philoſophers, to whom his language muſt, I am perſuaded, ſound very ſtrange. They would ſhow, by obſervation and experiment, that nothing of this kind has ever happened, and would ſay they had then proved that the expectation of its happening was very *unreaſonable*; but would think it a ſtrange abuſe of words to call it *nonſenſical*. To nonſenſe, as the term has generally been uſed hitherto, no ideas at all can be annexed, except ſuch as are inconſiſtent with

with one another; and we can form as clear an idea of lead *not* ſinking in water, as of its ſinking. What is really nonſenſe can never become ſenſe; but by miraculous power the laws of nature can be ſuſpended or reverſed.

To enlarge the province of this new principle of common ſenſe, Dr. Oſwald manifeſtly incroaches upon the province of reaſon in other inſtances. He expreſſes the greateſt poſſible ſurprize and indignation that divines ſhould have endeavoured 'to diſcover a medium to 'demonſtrate that we ought to worſhip 'God, to do juſtice to men, and to keep 'our paſſions and appetites within juſt 'and proper bounds,' p. 91. Upon this occaſion he ſays, as was quoted above, 'No demonſtration is of equal force with 'common ſenſe; and no confutation can 'ſerve the intereſt of truth ſo effectually 'as a plain conviction of nonſenſe; and 'therefore it was the buſineſs of divines 'and philoſophers to have recourſe to 'the

'the ſimple deciſion of common ſenſe on 'a ſubject ſo plain and important.'

I cannot help thinking, however, that it would anſwer a very good purpoſe both to define ſtrictly what we mean by *worſhiping God, doing juſtice to men*, and *bringing our paſſions within proper bounds;* and alſo that, when theſe propoſitions have been defined, intermediate and plainer propoſitions may be found, which will ſerve to ſhow the truth of the former. And ſuch proofs of theſe moral duties I think have been given by many writers, and I hope have not been impertinently alledged in my *Inſtitutes of natural and revealed religion*, vol. 1.

I am the more ſurprized at Dr. Oſwald's objections to the common language of logicians, as he himſelf diſtinguiſhes very well between ſuch propoſitions as are ſelf evident, and ſuch as are not. 'No man,' ſays he, p. 248, 'can be at a loſs to know 'propoſitions that are the object of com- 'mon

'mon ſenſe from thoſe that are not, and 'to determine with himſelf where he has, 'or has not a right to ſuſpend his judg-'ment. If the evidence of the propo-'ſition under conſideration flows from its 'relation to or connection with ſome 'other truth, he has no doubt a right to 'ſuſpend his judgment till he has inquired 'into that connexion and relation.'

Now ſurely the propoſition that *magi-ſtrates ought to be obeyed* depends upon this other propoſition, that *the good of the ſociety ought to be provided for*. Or if our author be an advocate for a natural and divine right, ſtill he muſt give ſome rea-ſon for it. If he reflect at all upon the ſubject, he will hardly maintain that ſuch a right is *ſelf evident*. This latter propo-ſition then, viz. that *the good of the ſtate ought to be conſulted*, may properly be urged in ſupport of the former, that ma-giſtrates ought to be obeyed. It is ſo much of an *argument*, that I dare ſay nei-ther our author, nor any other perſon, could

could possibly avoid it in discoursing on the subject.

Our author, indeed, admits of *a kind of demonstration* of primary truths, which arises from *comparing them with their opposite absurdities*; in consequence of which he says, p. 255, 'we shall believe them more 'cordially, and feel their influence more 'sensibly than we do. A real believer, he says, 'will not despise the well meant 'labours of those who have endeavoured 'to demonstrate the primary truths by 'reducing their opposites to absurdity; 'but knows that, without their help, he 'can, by a single thought, reduce these 'chimeras to the grossest of all absurdities, 'namely, to nonsense.' Though, therefore, it is *pardonable* to demonstrate the being and perfections of God, the necessity of obeying magistrates, &c. he advises us to spare ourselves that trouble, and with more magnanimity appeal at once to the great tribunal of common sense. An admirably short and decisive method

method truly! ſomething ſimilar to Defoe's *Short method with the Diſſenters;* with this difference, that Defoe was in jeſt, but Dr. Oſwald is in moſt ſerious earneſt.

Such is the force of common ſenſe; in my uſe of the word, that our author not only allows of reaſoning in others, but falls into downright reaſoning himſelf upon ſeveral ſubjects, which he had expreſsly exempted from the province of reaſoning, and in the very chapter in the title of which he diſclaims reaſoning.

'Lord Bolingbroke,' he ſays, vol. 2, p. 276, 'who contends ſo zealouſly for 'the being and providence of God, is no 'leſs zealous in decrying our natural 'notions of his moral perfections, and 'moral government, together with the 'expectation we have of an exact retri-'bution of our good and evil actions. 'But never was a great genius more ab-'ſurdly, or indeed more idly employed. 'For, in ſpite of all the arts of logic, of 'rhetoric, of bullying, and of canting, 'practiced by his Lordſhip, every one 'who believes there is a God will believe 'that he loves the right and hates the 'wrong; and expect, of courſe, that he 'will reward the one and puniſh the 'other.' Now is not Dr. Oſwald's ſuggeſting that God *loves the right and hates the wrong* a proper *argument*, to prove that he will reward the one and puniſh the other? Indeed, why did he uſe the word *therefore*, if he was not *arguing* and proving one thing by means of another? If this be not reaſoning, and in the neceſſary forms, I know not what is.

But, poſſibly, our author might think himſelf ſufficiently guarded againſt this objection by the manner in which he has expreſſed the title of this chapter, which is ingenious enough. 'To maintain, vol. 2, p. 276, 'a curious debate about a 'future judgment, when we ought to be 'preparing for ſo awful an event, is 'unpardonable folly.' The three next chap-

chapters have the title of '*The same sub-* '*ject continued.*'

The objection then is not to *arguments*, but to *curious arguments*. But how shall we distinguish curious debates from those that are not curious, and what does our author mean by *curious?* A word of so very vague a meaning is certainly very improperly used upon such an occasion as this. If I should be asked to point to a specimen of *curious reasoning*, I should name this very treatise of Dr. Oswald's.

But the propriety of the title of this same chapter is guarded in another curious manner. 'It is unpardonable folly,' he says, 'to maintain a curious debate 'about a future judgment, when we ought 'to be preparing for it.' But whoever denied that there was a time to *prepare* for a future event, as well as for *proving* that it will happen, and that these two ought not to interfere with one another? If he meant that we ought never to debate, but to be always preparing, it was unpardonable folly in him to write his treatife; in which he not only debates, but is the occafion of more debating, as the book I am now writing evidences.

I have defcanted a little upon the title of this one chapter, or rather of four chapters (which, by the way, is very aukward and confufed in point of method) in order to exhibit a fpecimen of our author's unfair and equivocal manner of writing throughout. By an artful choice of words he makes, upon all occafions, a fpecious harangue, when his pompous affertions are all the while either nugatory, or falfe.

As the greateft part of Dr. Ofwald's two volumes confifts of fuch writing as this, I fhall, for the more complete information of my reader concerning the nature of it, produce another example of his artfully adopting a mode of expreffion which cuts off all reply, except that of its being abfolutely trifling; while he is ufing all the pomp and

and parade of the moſt important obſervations.

'To ſtate the primary truths,' p. 315, 'in their native light and ſtrength, and in 'compariſon with their oppoſite falſities, 'and to ſhow, in the cleareſt, plaineſt 'manner, which ought to preponderate, was in juſtice due to the public. 'But to trace every conceit, of every 'bold projector, through all the windings 'of abſtruſe and ſophiſtical reaſoning, or 'to offer laborious and minute defences 'of truths which neither require nor ad'mit of any, was ill adviſed.'

I challenge our author to ſpecify the writers on whom this cenſure falls, viz. thoſe who have *traced every conceit of every bold projector through all the windings of abſtruſe and ſophiſtical reaſoning*, or who have *offered laborious and minute defences of truths which neither required nor admitted of any*. One would imagine, from reading Dr. Oſwald, that this egregious and laborious trifling had been univerſal

 with

with the infatuated friends of religion. But let our author name the men, and prove his charge; or be confidered as having given himfelf ridiculous airs, by cloathing mere calumny in rant.

Indeed, the exceptions which our author himfelf makes to his violent accufations will almoft amount to a full confutation of his declamatory abufe.

'It was no doubt proper,' he fays, p. 316, 'to detect the fcandalous fhuffling 'of Collins, to expofe the rambling con-'ceits of Lord Shaftefbury, the dangerous 'paradoxes of Mr. Hume, and the pre-'fumptuous boldnefs of Lord Boling-'broke. It might alfo be fit to take fome 'notice of the quibbles of inferior writers. 'But to engage the attention of a whole 'nation to a formal difpute between grave 'divines, and writers of this ftamp, about 'the truth of religion, as if this was a point 'yet unfettled, was a manner of proceeding 'much below the dignity of the fubject, 'and from which little good could be ex-'pected.

'pected. From the common effect produced on the minds of the multitude, 'by attending the pleading of lawyers in 'a contentious law suit, one might foretel the consequences of this ill judged 'measure.'

Now I really do not know to what kind of reasoning any of the defenders of christianity have had recourse, except such as was adopted in the controversies above referred to, and which our author allows to have been proper. And, exclusive of such controversies as he himself expressly approves, I challenge him to say when the *attention of any whole nation was ever engaged to a formal dispute between grave divines about the truth of religion, as if it was a point yet unsettled.* This assertion, I will venture to say, was made absolutely at random, and has no foundation in truth. It is a mere rhetorical flourish, in support of a piece of miserable sophistry.

Our author farther allows, vol. 2, p. 78, that 'the disciples of Manes were intitled 'to ſatisfaction, becauſe,' as he curiouſly enough expreſſes it, 'they *founded on* '*realities*.' He adds, 'but it is below 'the dignity of divines or philoſophers to 'fight with chimeras. Theſe antient 'heretics had not the boldneſs of modern 'theoriſts, who ſcruple not to reſolve 'natural and moral evil into the divine 'will; but from the ſame averſion which 'all guilty perſons have of bringing the 'charge home to themſelves, they fancied 'themſelves under the neceſſity of hav'ing recourſe to two gods, the authors 'of all that is good or evil in the world.'

Not to remark upon our author's taking it for granted that all Neceſſarians are unbelievers (though the very beſt of all the defences of chriſtianity has been written by a Neceſſarian) I ſhall only aſk, whether all who object to religion and chriſtianity do not pretend to found their objections on *realities*, as well as Manes.

The remainder of the paragraph quoted above is not leſs curious, and of a piece with

with the reſt of the treatiſe. ' This groſs ' error,' viz. that of Manes ' is, however, ' long ſince extinct, and the friends of ' religion can be under no obligation to ' prove the unity of God, till at leaſt ' ſome one appear who can ſay, with a ' good conſcience, that he ſuſpects that ' there are more than one, to whom we ' owe that worſhip and obedience which is ' due, in return for his being and pre- ' ſervation; and till he aſſign ſome ' plauſible reaſon for his ſuſpicion.' p. 79.

But can there be no propriety or advantage in reviewing the errors of paſt ages, and in the confutation of them? May we not hope, by that means, to prevent a relapſe into them? Can we be too well eſtabliſhed in truths of great importance? Beſides, with reſpect to this very queſtion, of the *unity of God*, has not the church of Rome, the church of England, and even the church of Scotland, more objects of ſupreme worſhip than one?

I would

I would alſo aſk, what the word *plauſi-ble* has to do in this buſineſs. If an error be *actually* embraced, and ſpreads; muſt I defer the combating of it till ſome *grand jury*, appointed for the purpoſe, ſhall vote that it is a plauſible one? Had theſe preliminaries been requiſite, it is not certain that I ſhould have been permitted to anſwer Dr. Oſwald.

I ſhall produce but one inſtance more of our author's complaints of the conduct of chriſtian divines, who have judged and acted differently from himſelf; becauſe, *for once*, he names his man. 'Had Dr. 'Clarke,' p. 151, 'employed his natural 'good ſenſe, which was not inferior to 'his learning, in ſetting in a true and full 'light all the ſhameful abſurdities of thoſe 'who believe there is a God, and behave 'as if there was none, he would have 'done more ſervice to the intereſts of 'truth, than can be done by a thouſand 'demonſtrations.'

But

But why may it not be of ſervice to ſet in a ſtrong light the abſurdity of not believing or affecting not to believe that there is a God, as well as of not acting in a manner agreeable to that belief? The latter is certainly as obvious, and therefore is as little neceſſary to be inſiſted upon as the former. But ſo great is our author's averſion to *reaſoning*, that a man muſt not touch upon the former, however neceſſary, becauſe ſomething like *argument*, *proof* and *demonſtration* may be wanted; whereas on the latter of theſe topics a man may declaim as long as he pleaſes, writing as Dr. Oſwald does, without any reaſoning at all.

Laſtly, our author very much miſrepreſents the conduct of the *ſacred writers*, in order to favour his ſyſtem, and to decry reaſoning. 'The inſpired writers do 'not offer any proof of the being and 'perfections of God. They tell us that 'the inviſible things of him are clearly 'ſeen from the things which he has 'made, &c.—but never enter into trains

'of

'of reaſoning, to eſtabliſh a truth that is 'too obvious to admit of any proof.' Vol. 2, p. 51, 52.

But how do any divines pretend to prove the inviſible power of God otherwiſe than by the viſible effects of it; at leaſt I never had recourſe to any other argument, and yet I imagine that I have reaſoned on the ſubject. See my Inſtitutes, vol. 1.

Perhaps our author may think to eſcape my animadverſions, by ſaying that, though the ſacred writers do reaſon, they do not enter into *trains of reaſoning* on the ſubject. But whether a man uſes trains of reaſoning or not, or whether the trains be longer or ſhorter is not the queſtion; but whether they reaſon at all. In my opinion our author may find both excellent reaſoning and even long trains of reaſoning on the being, perfections, and providence of God in various parts of the books of ſcripture, as in the book of Job, the Pſalms, and the Prophets. In my my opinion Paul reaſoned very cloſely on this ſubject in his diſcourſe before the Athenian Areopagites. See Acts xvii. But the ſacred writers had no occaſion to prove the being or perfections of God to thoſe who admitted them, which was generally the caſe with thoſe to whom, or for whom they wrote.

---

## SECTION VI.

### *Of Dr.* Oſwald's *refutation of the argument in proof of the* being of a God.

THERE is no ſubject on which Dr. Oſwald declaims ſo frequently, or with ſo much vehemence, and ſeeming ſatisfaction to himſelf, as on the want of judgment in divines, in reaſoning concerning the *being of a God;* which he always ſpeaks of as 'too obvious and ſacred a truth to be ſubjected to the reaſonings of men, and that too much en-

' courage-

'courragement has been given to the ca-
'vils of ſceptics by entering into reaſon-
'ing about it.' Theſe propoſitions are the titles of two ſeparate chapters in his ſecond volume, p. 50 and 57.

In the latter of theſe chapters he even openly aſſumes the character of an atheiſt, and undertakes a complete refutation of the ſtanding argument for the being of a God, in order to ſhew that it is incapable of any proper *proof;* but that the propoſition, being nevertheleſs true, muſt be admitted on the ſole authority of common ſenſe; not conſidering that if this new principle of common ſenſe ſhould ever be exploded, he has no reſource left, but muſt in good earneſt profeſs himſelf an atheiſt. And thus, like the dog in the fable, by catching at a ſhadow, he will have loſt the ſubſtance. Now, as I ſhould be very ſorry for ſuch a cataſtrophe, I ſhall go over the ſeveral ſteps of this demonſtration along with Dr. Oſwald; in order to convince him, that, notwithſtanding his confident objections,

jections, it is a very good one, and will bear the strictest examination.

'No process of reasoning,' says Dr. Oswald, vol. 2, p. 57, 'can be employed 'in favour of this capital truth, that will 'not be found either false or frivolous; 'or if the premises are admitted to proof, 'there can be no just conclusion. The 'premises are these, a work that indicates 'design must be ascribed to an intelligent 'author. The world is a work that in'dicates design,' &c.

From these premises, each of which Dr. Oswald allows to be just, though not demonstrable, I think it may be clearly proved that *the world must be ascribed to an intelligent author*, which is what we mean by the term *God*. If the conclusion be allowed to be fairly drawn from the premises, which Dr. Oswald does not deny, the argument is certainly complete, whether we proceed any farther, viz. to prove the truth of the premises or not. To this, however, our author gives no atten-

attention; but only ſays it is impoſſible to prove the premiſes. Let us conſider then, in what manner he pretends that neither of theſe premiſes can be proved, ſo that an unbeliever may be juſtified in witholding his aſſent to them, and conſequently from the concluſion that is drawn from them.

'A work that indicates deſign muſt be 'aſcribed to an intelligent author.'

This is an abſtract propoſition, to which, if the terms of it be defined, I will venture to ſay that no man can poſſibly withhold his aſſent, being really identical and ſelf-evident. To invalidate this, or rather to evade it, our author abſolutely *changes* it, and ſubſtitutes another in its place. For, from an abſtract and *univerſal*, he makes it a *particular* propoſition; aſſerting as the reverſe of it, that this particular work, viz. *this world, bears no marks of deſign;* in ſupport of which he alledges the trite atheiſtical ſuppoſition of the poſſibility of its having been produced

duced by the *concourſe of atoms*. 'By 'repeated throws of dice,' he ſays, vol. 2, p. 59, 'one may caſt up any number 'called for, within a given time; and 'therefore any poſſible ſtate of nature 'may reſult from unlimited revolutions 'of matter.'

Not to ſay that this does not amount to a ſhadow of an objection to the truth of a propoſition, which only aſſerts that a work which *actually does* indicate deſign is to be aſcribed to an intelligent author; which, by ſuppoſition, excludes all idea of chance, it may certainly be ſaid, on the behalf of the being of a God, that let atoms revolve, *ad infinitum*, and move without a mover, nothing can reſult from it but new *combinations*, and *poſitions*. For *powers*, ſuch as thoſe of attraction, repulſion, magnetiſm, electricity, &c. could never be gained by it; there being no conceivable or poſſible connection between ſuch a revolution, and the acquiſition of any ſuch powers. It is poſſible that the ingenuity of Dr. Oſwald may ſuggeſt ſomething to an atheiſt in anſwer to this, but I own I cannot. And yet, as if the believer could make no reply to this objection, which is both miſplaced and frivolous, he concludes that he had ſufficiently invalidated the force of this *major* propoſition, and proceeds with great confidence to attack the minor, viz. that

'The world is a work that indicates 'deſign.'

Here, after acknowledging, p. 61, 'that it is eaſy to ſhow them (atheiſts) a 'connection of parts and unity of deſign, 'which they cannot gainſay;' yet he maintains that, 'becauſe they can point 'out ſome ſtrange and uncouth appear- 'ances, which we cannot explain, they 'have a right to withhold their aſſent, 'if the caſe is to be determined by reaſon, 'and not by the authority of common 'ſenſe. But ſurely, after admitting 'deſign in *many things*, they cannot poſſi- 'bly withhold their aſſent to *thoſe things*

'having

'having an intelligent author, whatever 'they may do with reſpect to the reſt.'

If, for inſtance, it be undeniable, that the formation of the eye, and of the light, which ſo admirably correſpond to one another, and to the purpoſe of giving us notices of diſtant objects, is an excellent *contrivance;* it is plain that there muſt have been a *contriver*, or an intelligent author of *that part* of our conſtitution, though there ſhould be other parts of the ſame ſyſtem, the ſpleen, for inſtance, the uſes of which we could not explain. So that it appears to me, that the propoſition is completely proved, according to the ſtricteſt forms of logic.

But our author ſays, 'You may unriddle many difficulties, and give ſatiſfaction to ſeveral objections. You may 'do more. By careful inſpection, you 'can ſhow, to the ſatisfaction of the 'ſceptic, that what appeared irregularity 'is regularity in the higheſt degree; that 'ſeeming diſcord is harmony not un-

'derſtood, and that a ſeeming blemiſh 'is a beauty in the works of God; but 'you will not ſilence him. You have 'ſomething farther to explain, and ſome-'thing farther ſtill, and cannot give a 'full anſwer to his objections until you 'explain the whole, and that you cannot 'do. Good ſenſe requires that he ſhould 'be contented with leſs ſatisfaction, but 'he demands *proof*, and as you have 'undertaken it, you muſt give it without 'reſerve or limitation.'

The propoſition, however, propoſes no ſuch thing. It only aſſerts that this world muſt have had an intelligent author. So that if I prove that *any thing* in the world neceſſarily requires ſuch an author, which Dr. Oſwald himſelf, in the character of a ſceptic, allows, I have fully proved all that I propoſed. I will venture to ſay, that no perſon, who ever propoſed the ſtricteſt demonſtration of the being of God, ever thought of any thing elſe; and I even challenge Dr. Oſwald to name any atheiſt who expected more.

If

If a man ſhould be ſo fooliſh as to give out that he could explain all the phenomena of nature, which he certainly could not do, and ſhould acknowledge that he had not demonſtrated the being of a God till he had done it, I do not ſee how *good ſenſe* ſhould help a man to ſee that he had fulfilled his promiſe, when it was evident to *reaſon* that he had not done it. If, therefore, a man advances no more than he can prove, which is ſufficient for the demonſtration of the being of a God, an appeal may as ſafely be made to *reaſon*, as to any thing bearing the name of *common ſenſe*, or any other name that admits of *evidence without proof*. As, on the other hand, if he advances more than he can prove, I do not think that there is any power in human nature that can oblige us to ſay that he had done what he himſelf acknowledges he could not do.

At the concluſion, however, of all this miſerable quibbling and ſophiſtry, our author ſums up his chapter with the airs of an acknowledged conqueror. 'Whe-

'ther the ſceptic is actuated by imper-
'tinent curioſity, a ſpirit of contradiction,
'or a yet worſe principle, it muſt be
'owned that, as a diſputant, he has a
'right to inſiſt on his demand; and, on
'being refuſed, to withhold his aſſent;
'which he can do with the more eaſe,
'and with a much better grace, in the
'courſe of a diſpute, than he could have
'done, if you had ſubmitted the truth to
'his judgment, by a ſimple appeal.' That is, if I *beg the queſtion*, he may, as a *favour*, condeſcend to grant it.

'It is ſurprizing,' continues our author,
'that this inconvenience attending the
'method of argumentation ſhould have
'been ſo long overlooked by ſo many
'friends of religion, diſtinguiſhed by their
'good ſenſe, as well as by their learning.
'Yet any one may recollect ſimilar in-
'ſtances of men of good underſtanding,
'diſappointing themſelves in common life,
'by too great eagerneſs to prove truths
'too obvious to admit of proof or de-
'monſtration.'

But

But what had eſcaped not only the *learning*, but, what is much more, the *good ſenſe* of all preceding ages, has been luckily diſcovered by our author.——To conclude this ſection with ſerioufneſs. I know no parallel to ſuch wretched ſophiſtry and conceit. And that any *friend of religion* ſhould thus lend weapons to the common adverſaries, and in their name, challenge all the powers of reaſon, certainly would not have gained credit before the publication of this work of Dr. Oſwald's. Such are the happy fruits of diſcarding reaſon, and ſubſtituting this new common ſenſe in its place. And yet this is the man, who, upon all occaſions, and from the beginning of his two volumes to the end of them, ridicules and inſults the greateſt maſters of argumentation.

'Can you tell me,' ſays he, p. 375, 'whence it comes to paſs, that our celebrated divines and philoſophers blunder 'ſo groſsly in an art to which they are ſo 'much devoted?' But before a man had affected this contempt of reaſoning, he ſhould certainly have known *what it was;* which appears not to have been the caſe with Dr. Oſwald. I have ſtudied, and I have taught logic, but in no ſcholar's exerciſe did I ever ſee ſuch marks of a total ignorance of the plaineſt rules of it, as in Dr. Oſwald's critical examination of the argument for the being of God; and it is evident that in him common ſenſe has not ſupplied the place of logic, though he boaſts of it's doing infinitely more.

## SECTION VII.

*Of the application of Common ſenſe to various diſquiſitions in* Morals *and* Theology.

WHEN the idea of this new ſenſe was firſt ſtarted, it had the appearance of ſomething new and whimſical, indeed, but it threatened nothing; ſeeming to be only a new method of explaining the manner in which we give our aſſent to ſelf-evident propoſitions; and, provided the propoſitions were really ſelf evident, it ſignified nothing in practice by what means we evince them to be ſo.

Going thus backwards, into the obſcure regions of *Metaphyſics*, could do no great harm, and might prove an innocent amuſement to many perſons who had nothing better to do, or to thoſe who choſe to relax from more important ſtudies. But when this new power, after thus ſecuring its retreat backwards, begins to advance

advance forwards, into the regions of *ſcience*, *philoſophy*, and *life*, ſuperſeding reaſoning wherever it comes, we begin to mark its progreſs with more attention: for we muſt not ſuffer her invaſion of the right of another. Accordingly I have endeavoured to repreſs the inroads which this new power has made on the *frontiers* of morals and theology; and now I muſt ſhow what attempts ſhe has made to penetrate into the *interior parts* of the country.

To drop this alluſion, which I am not able to carry much farther, I propoſe, in this laſt ſection, to exhibit to my reader the ſummary proceſs by which our author treats ſeveral intricate and important queſtions; as *the ſpring of action in the deity*, *the diſtinction between the faculties of men and brutes*, and the doctrines, or pretended doctrines, of the *divinity of Chriſt*, *atonement*, *the new birth*, and *predeſtination*, with other ſmaller matters. None of theſe ſubjects, which have been thought to be very difficult, and which have

have exercifed the genius of the ableft men in all nations, occafion the leaft difficulty to Dr. Ofwald. His common fenfe knows no difference of queftions, but decides with equal *quicknefs*, *clearnefs*, and *indubitable certainty*, on every thing that you fhall bring before it. Hear then in what manner our author decides the long and well debated queftion concerning the *fpring of action in the deity*.

'The learned of our day,' vol. 2, p. 156, 'will have us to think that happinefs, mere happinefs, is the ultimate 'end and object of the divine govern-'ment.——They confidently affirm that 'a being completely happy in himfelf 'could have no other end in bringing 'creatures into exiftence, than to make 'them happy. But this is unpardonable 'rafhnefs. For if the fole end of bring-'ing creatures into being was to make 'them happy, then they could not be in 'pain or mifery for a fingle moment; be-'caufe the fupreme ruler could not be 'difappointed of his end in one fingle 'inftance,

'inftance, or for one moment of time. 'Plans formed by beings of limited ca- 'pacity may fail in the execution, but no 'defect can be imputed to him whofe un- 'derftanding is infinite, and whofe power 'without control. This hypothefis, there- 'fore, muft be fundamentally wrong. It 'is plain,' vol. 2, p. 157, 'God does not 'all that is poffible to be done to make his 'creatures happy.'

Having thus, contrary to his cuftom, condefcended to overturn by reafon a fcheme that was founded on reafon, he eftablifhes another, and, as far as I know, a fcheme intirely his own, which cannot fail to recommend it to my reader, on the foundation of common fenfe.

'Common fenfe,' vol. 2, p. 157, 'will 'hardly authorize weak mortals to fix 'the ultimate end and object of the 'divine government, but the greateft 'poffible increafe of moral worth feems 'beft to correfpond to appearances, and 'to the dignity of the fup reme ruler, and, 'probably,

'probably, was meant in the laſt age by 'the glory of God, and is now exchanged 'for the happineſs of the creature, by 'thoſe who favour a more lax theology, 'the tendency of which error is to bring 'down virtue to the rank of a mean or 'ſubordinate end; the place it always 'held with hypocrites and villains of all 'kinds, who regard it no farther than it 'ſerves their purpoſe.'

Here we ſee our author not depending intirely upon the force of his principle of common ſenſe, but willing to take a little *indirect advantage*, by repreſenting his opponents as perſons who favour a lax theology, and who regard virtue no farther than it ſerves their purpoſes. But not to digreſs.

'It is impoſſible,' vol. 2, p. 111, 'that 'the deity ſhould have any other object 'of his government beſides the exerciſe 'and enjoyment of his own adorable per-'fections.—He makes the good happy, 'and the bad wretched, not from any

'ſuch

'ſuch political reaſons as influence human 'government, but from the eſſential per- 'fections of his nature.'

One would think that the ſcheme which our author adopts, viz. the greateſt poſſible increaſe of moral worth (which differs materially from the ſcheme of *rectitude* propoſed by Dr. Balguy, or that of *wiſdom* by Mr. Grove) was liable to the very ſame objection which he thought unanſwerable with reſpect to the ſcheme of benevolence. For it is as evident that God has not made all his intelligent creatures completely *virtuous*, as that he has not made them completely *happy*; eſpecially as our author will not deny that the divine being might, if he had thought proper, have influenced the minds of his creatures, or have originally formed them ſo, that nothing could have overpowered their inclination to virtue. But common ſenſe, it ſeems, declares that, though this objection was ſufficient to overturn the ſcheme of benevolence, it is impertinence to urge it againſt this new ſcheme of our author's.

author's. So eaſily does this principle decide where there ſeems to be nothing to determine the judgment; in which it bears a wonderful reſemblance to the *ſelf determining power* in man. But hear the oracle.

'Whether God,' vol. 2, p. 342, 'might 'not have ordered things, ſo that men 'would have been laid under the ſame 'neceſſity of regulating themſelves by 'the laws of nature, is an impertinent 'queſtion, becauſe we know he will not.'

However, to give us ſome little help to our conceptions, beſides this authoritative determination of common ſenſe, our author tranſports us into the inviſible world of ſpirits, and gives us a proſpect that cannot fail to demonſtrate the unſpeakable preference of his ſcheme above that of benevolence.

After deſcribing a good man having *broke looſe from this cumberſome fleſh*, and *eſcaped the vanities of life*, and being

*brought*

*brought into the preſenſe of God*, with what he feels then, and what he finds he has to do afterwards, he ſays, vol. 2, p. 177, 'This is a proſpect we muſt al'low to be grand; and whether this, or 'a ſucceſſion of pleaſurable ſenſations, is 'the moſt worthy of the ultimate end and 'object of the ſupreme ruler, may be ſub'mitted to every one who is endued with 'the judgment and ſpirit of man.'

Let us now appeal to this new oracle on the ſubject of a much controverted point of divinity, about which profane reaſon might have buſied itſelf to no purpoſe, and which has much embarraſſed many chriſtian divines, eſpecially thoſe who have received certain emoluments from religious eſtabliſhments, on the condition of maintaining the ſame faith with the *all-wiſe* founders of thoſe happy eſtabliſhments. I now mean the knotty queſtion of the *equality of the ſon of God with his father*. Now, by the help of this omnipotent common ſenſe, we are able to keep clear of all difficulties, and even to ſteer evenly

evenly between the two oppoſite rocks of the *creation*, and *no-creation* of the ſon of God.

'The ſon of God derives life from the 'Father in a manner totally different from 'creation, and which we neither under-'ſtand, nor have any occaſion to inquire 'into, any farther than is neceſſary to aſ-'ſure us, that he is of a rank as much 'ſuperior to created beings, as he has 'obtained a more excellent name than 'they.' Vol. 2, p. 128.

Now, by the way, I rather ſuſpect that our author's philoſophy and ſyſtematical theology do not perfectly tally. The Aſſembly's catechiſm, which I preſume our author has ſubſcribed, and by which he holds his church preferment, ſays that the three perſons in the godhead are of *the ſame ſubſtance, equal in power and glory*, which I ſhould think to be hardly conſiſtent with the notion of the ſon deriving life from the Father; however it may be *ſoftened*, or rather *obſcured*, by ſaying that this derivation is ſomething eſſentially different from *creation*. But we may take it for granted that ſo *pious* a man as Dr. Oſwald could not poſſibly *prevaricate* in a matter of this nature, eſpecially after his own ſolemn declaration on the ſubject.

'We appeal to common ſenſe, and 'defy them to offer a ſhadow of reaſon, 'why the man who prevaricates in reli- 'ligion ſhould not be as much the object 'of contempt and abhorrence, as he who 'prevaricates on any other ſubject of im- 'portance.' Vol. 2, p. 115. I ſhould be glad, however, if our author would condeſcend to clear up the conſiſtency of his conduct in this caſe, for the ſatisfaction of ſome whoſe common ſenſe is not ſo nice and diſtinguiſhing as his, and who cannot ſplit ſo fine a hair.

With reſpect to the doctrine of *atonement*, our author's common ſenſe decides likewiſe in favour of orthodoxy, which is a great happineſs, as it ſaves him the trouble

trouble of conſidering and anſwering a great number of ſhrewd objections to that ſuppoſed doctrine of ſcripture.

Speaking of the diſpenſation of the goſpel, he ſays, p. 50, 'Meſſengers were 'diſpatched to the different nations, calling upon them to forſake their vices and 'impieties, and to return to God, who 'was willing to receive them to favour, 'through the mediation of that divine 'perſon; who, having expiated their 'guilt by his death, has aſcended into 'heaven.' He calls Chriſt, vol. 2, p. 98, 'a perſon of the higheſt dignity, who, by 'a courſe of unparalleled obedience, has '*merited*, in the ſtricteſt ſenſe of the word, 'favours of various kinds for his adherents, which in no conſiſtency with wiſdom, equity, or juſtice, could otherwiſe 'be conferred upon them. Can we ſuppoſe,' ſays he, vol. 2, p. 161, 'that a 'good God would ſuffer a perſon of ſuch 'an amiable character, and one ſo near and 'dear to him, to undergo ſuch exquiſite

'ſufferings, if juſtice did not make it ne-
'ceſſary?'

The doctrines of *divine influence*, and the *new birth* have given much exerciſe to ſome inquiſitive minds, but as they give no trouble to our author, he wonders that any body elſe ſhould have found the leaſt difficulty in them. Common ſenſe can ſolve theſe difficulties, and much greater.

'One cannot help ſmiling,' ſays our author, 'at the pitiful ſhifts which the 'pretenders to learning go into, to ex-'tricate themſelves from the embarraſſ-'ment they are under with reſpect to 'the operation of the Holy Ghoſt, and 'the new birth, which to a man of true 'judgment, creates no difficulty at all,' vol. 2, p. 137. Then, comparing this ſupernatural influence to the *light of the ſun*, he ſays, 'Why then, may not he, 'with equal eaſe, and with equal ſafety 'to the order of nature, and without the

'leaſt

'least infringement of any of its laws, pro-
'duce a total change of sentiments and
'inclinations, with new habits of thinking
'and acting, in those who resign them-
'selves to his influence, and conform
'themselves to his direction. If this
'subject were explained by the same
'rules of good sense, and true philoso-
'phy, which are employed on subjects of
'far less consequence, the *new birth*
'would be equally intelligible with any
'other of the productions of nature we
'seem to be best acquainted with.'

Hitherto our author's common sense has always happened to steer him pretty nearly into the safe and comfortable harbour of orthodoxy, but with respect to the doctrine concerning the *power of man to do the will of God,* I am afraid it will appear to have driven him quite wide of it. For if I have any knowledge of scholastic divinity, Dr. Oswald's doctrine on this subject is the very reverse of what the Scotch ministers are obliged to ſubſcribe, as well as to that of the church of England.

'Take one of the vulgar aſide,' vol. 2, p. 208, 'and point out to him *ſome* duties 'he neglects, and ſome vices he indulges. '—He will acknowledge the fact, but 'will conclude that till God work it in 'him he can do nothing. This,' ſays he, p. 208, 'they are taught to ſay.' And ſo, if I be not greatly miſtaken, Dr. Oſwald himſelf is under an obligation, equivalent to the moſt ſolemn of all oaths, to teach them.

'To alledge the neceſſity,' p. 212, 'of 'an interpoſition which we have no reaſon 'to expect, and which one in an hundred 'is not favoured with, is a heinous im'piety: for it amounts to nothing leſs 'than a declaration, that the ſupreme 'being looks on, and ſees ninety nine of 'a hundred periſh for want of an inter'poſition, which is neceſſary to deter'mine them to do the right and ſhun the 'wrong.'

This

This is certainly very ſound Arminian doctrine, but very unſound Calviniſm. If our author holds his Scotch living, I hope he will explain, in his next, how he can do this, and keep clear of a dangerous refinement, and *prevarication in matters of religion.* Let him take care that this *common ſenſe* do not a little interfere with *common honeſty*, and chriſtian ſincerity.

The difference between the *intellectual faculties of men and brutes* has occaſioned a good deal of difficulty both to philoſophers and divines; but on this ſubject our author is equally clear and deciſive as on all the others on which he has favoured us with his opinion. In ſhort, it is Common ſenſe that is *the characteriſtic of rationality. Every individual of the human race* has it, ideots excepted.

'If,' ſays our author, p. 186, 'we
'know any thing at all of the ſpecific
'difference between our underſtanding
'and that of inferior animals, it muſt con-

'sist in our having perceptions of truth 'which are imperceptible to them. Inferior animals,' p. 185, 'fly things of 'hurtful appearance, and pursue objects 'of pleasure and convenience, with a sagacity and earnestness, as if they really 'knew those powers in nature by which 'they may be profited or hurt. But that 'they do not know them in the manner 'we do; and, indeed, that they can have 'no idea of them at all appears from 'hence, that they never make the least 'attempt to employ those powers in their 'favour. There are numberless occasions,' ib. 'on which inferior animals 'could relieve themselves from danger 'and from death, if they had the least 'notion of many powers in nature which 'they could easily lay hold of. It is 'worthy of notice,' he says, p. 183, 'that 'brutes never thrust one another over 'precipices, into ponds, or rivers, or into 'fire. They may do it by accident, but 'never through mirth, or malice, as children do; because they have not those 'ideas of the laws of nature which chil-

'dren

'dren have. Who doubts,' p. 186, 'that 'many of the inferior animals, under deep 'provocation, would burn houſes, and 'do other dreadful acts of miſchief, if 'they had the leaſt idea of power in fire 'to conſume cumbuſtibles?'

Our author does not give himſelf the trouble to anſwer many objections, taking the eaſy method of treating them with contempt, as things that are, in their own nature, altogether impertinent, or I could mention ſeveral. Dogs may not have a fancy for puſhing one another into ponds, or into the fire, thinking perhaps there may be no great diverſion in it, but they mouthe and tumble one another about in a very pretty, and ingenious manner, juſt as if they knew as much of the laws of nature as relate to biting and tumbling; and ſome animals of the monkey tribe both divert themſelves and plague others, ſeemingly, with as perfect a knowledge of the natural powers of various inſtruments which they make uſe of for that purpoſe, as any unlucky young boy

in

in the world. As far as I ſee, brutes both judge and reaſon as properly as we do, as far as their ideas extend. But I mean not to diſcuſs any of theſe deep ſubjects, but only make ſuch obſervations as may tend to illuſtrate the ſentiments of my author.

The laſt article I ſhall mention (and I do not know whether Dr. Oſwald, my reader, or myſelf, is moſt pleaſed that I have got to the laſt article) is a very ſmall one indeed, but nothing can properly be called inconſiderable that relates to this moſt wonderful new diſcovered faculty of the human mind. So the moſt trifling cuſtom of a new diſcovered people engages more attention than the moſt ſolemn and important ones of our old neighbours. And though our author does not, in this caſe, mention any obligation he was under to his principle of common ſenſe, it might poſſibly have been of ſome indirect uſe to him in the diſcovery.

Moſt perſons who have any reſpect to religion, aſk a bleſſing on their meat, eſpecially when they ſit down to dine in a ſocial manner; and perhaps they may think they know the reaſon of this cuſtom; but I am now authorized to inform them that they are much miſtaken, and that they are not quite ſo wiſe as they fancy themſelves to be. In proof of this hear our author.

'There may be ſomething in man's 'conſtitution which deſtroys the nutritive 'quality of bread,, and may turn it into 'poiſon, which is a good philoſophical 'account of the common practice of aſk- 'ing a bleſſing on our food,' p. 372.

Having now dined very plentifully at the expence of our author, I thank him, for myſelf and my readers, for the entertainment he has given us. And that he may make his own epilogue, I ſhall conclude with what he ſays of the greatneſs of his ſcheme, and his hopes of ſucceſs in it. And to ſhew my readineſs to adopt my author's ſentiments, as far as I poſſibly can, I beg my reader would fancy to himſelf

ſelf that as ſoon as Dr. Oſwald has repeated the following ſentences, I alſo ſtand up, and, *mutatis mutandis,* repeat them audibly after him.

'I hope the public will take in good 'part,' p. 390, 'this effort I have made 'to check a folly which has retarded the 'progreſs of knowledge in all ages, and 'threatened the preſent age with a per-'verſion of judgment ſimilar to what 'prevailed in that period, when, as Mr. 'Pope ſays,

Faith, Goſpel, all ſeem'd made to be diſputed,
And none had ſenſe enough to be confuted.

'It is not poſſible', ſays he to his friend, p. 349, 'to give at once a new and op-'poſite turn to men's way of thinking'; but 'as I hope to ſatisfy your ſcruples in a 'little time, ſo I believe that in due time 'the bulk of mankind may be brought 'to a juſt way of thinking on this ſub-'ject.'

THE

THE

# APPENDIX.

THE

# APPENDIX.

## NUMBER I.

*Of the resemblance between the doctrine of* Common sense, *and the Principles of* Dr. Price's Review *of the questions and difficulties in morals.*

I Have mentioned my surprise that none of the authors on whom I have been animadverting should seem to have heard of *Dr. Hartley's Observations on man*, except Dr. Beattie, who appears not to have understood him, and who pays him the trifling compliment of an *ingenious but fanciful author*. I must also express my surprise, though not in the same degree, that none of them should have mentioned *Dr. Price's Review of the*

*the principal queſtions and difficulties in morals*, which was publiſhed in 1758; and which, both with reſpect to the theory of the mind, and the practical application of it, contains all that is original, and that has the appearance of being juſt and uſeful in any of them.

This writer, whoſe ſuperiority to Dr. Reid, Dr. Beattie, or Dr. Oſwald, is exceedingly manifeſt, maintains that the *underſtanding* is the ſource of many of our moſt important ſimple ideas; as that of *the neceſſary connection of events in nature*, the *vis inertiæ of matter*, *ſubſtance*, *duration*, *ſpace*, *infinity*, *neceſſity*, *equality*, *identity*, *contingency*, *poſſibility*, *power*, *and cauſation*, &c. and more eſpecially to this ſource he refers our *ideas of moral right and wrong*, and of *moral obligation*. It is, he obſerves, of the eſſence of theſe ideas to imply ſomething *true or falſe* of an object, and that they by no means denote the manner in which we are *affected* by it; ſo that they cannot with any propriety be referred to that part of our

con-

constitution which has hitherto been distinguished by the appellation of *sense*.

This scheme has all the flattering advantages of the new doctrine of common sense, without the capital inconveniencies attending it. Like this scheme, it cuts off, if it be admitted, (and without this no scheme can have any operation or effect) all objections to primary moral truths, resting them on a simple appeal to the faculty of *intuition*; and refusing to reason upon a subject which is maintained to be as evident as the truth of the geometrical postulatum, that *if equal things be taken from equal things the remainders will be equal*. But this philosopher had more good sense than to load his scheme with the belief of the real existence of the external world; and he is more especially careful to keep intirely clear of every thing that can represent our ideas of virtue as *arbitrary* and *precarious*, which is the necessary consequence of this new scheme.

If the ideas of moral right and wrong, &c. be perceived by a *ſenſe*, it depends upon our arbitrary conſtitution that we conceive of them as we do, or whether we perceive them at all; and we have no method whatever of inveſtigating whether they have any foundation in the abſolute *nature of things*. Whereas by making moral ideas the object of the *underſtanding* or intellect, *as ſuch*, the principles of morality become part of the ſyſtem of *neceſſary*, *eternal*, and *unalterable truth*, perceived by the divine being, as by ourſelves, but altogether independent of his will, as well as of all other beings, and things whatſoever; as much ſo as the truth of the *poſtulatum* above mentioned, or of the propoſition that *two and two make four*.

To exhibit as diſtinctly as poſſible this original ſcheme of Dr. Price's, with as much of the evidence of it as I can find expreſſed, in a ſhort compaſs, by the author himſelf, I ſhall preſent my reader with

with the following extracts from his very elaborate work.

'I cannot help wondering,' p. 48, 'that, 'in inquiring into the original of our 'ideas, the *underſtanding*, which, though 'not firſt in time, is the moſt important 'ſource of our ideas, ſhould have been 'overlooked. It has, indeed, been al-'ways conſidered as the ſource of *know-'ledge*; but it ſhould have been more at-'tended to, that, as the ſource of know-'ledge, it is likewiſe the ſource of *new 'ideas*, and that it cannot be one of theſe 'without being the other.'

'The various kinds of *agreement* and '*diſagreement* between our ideas, which, 'Mr. Locke ſays, is its office to diſcover 'and trace, are ſo many new ſimple ideas, 'of which it muſt itſelf have been the 'original. Thus when it conſiders the 'two angles made by a right line, ſtand-'ing in any direction on another, and 'perceives the *agreement* between them 'and two right angles, what is this *agree-*

'*ment* beſides their *equality?* And is not 'the idea of this equality a new ſimple 'idea, derived from the underſtanding, 'wholly different from that of the two 'angles compared, and repreſenting ſelf-'evident truth.'

'In much the ſame manner in other 'caſes, knowledge and intuition ſuppoſe 'ſomewhat perceived or diſcovered in 'their objects, denoting ſimple ideas, to 'which themſelves gave riſe. This is 'true of our ideas of *proportion,* of our 'ideas of *identity* and *diverſity, exiſtence,* '*connection, cauſe* and *effect, power, poſſi-* '*bility* and *impoſſibility,* and of our ideas 'of *moral right and wrong.* The firſt 'concerns *quantity,* the laſt *actions,* the 'reſt *all things.* They comprehend the 'moſt conſiderable part of what we can 'deſire to *know* of things, and are the ob-'jects of almoſt all reaſonings and diſ-'quiſitions.'

'It is therefore eſſential to the under-'ſtanding to be the fountain of new

'ideas.

'ideas. As bodily ſight diſcovers to us 'the qualities of outward viſible objects, 'ſo does the underſtanding, which is the 'eye of the mind, and infinitely more 'ſubtle and penetrating, diſcover to us 'the qualities of intelligible objects; and 'thus, in a like ſenſe with the former, 'becomes the inlet of new ideas.'

The whole of what Dr. Beattie and Dr. Oſwald have written about the neceſſity of acquieſcing in primary truths, and on the inutility and inſufficiency of reaſoning in many caſes, is ſo fully expreſſed by Dr. Price, that one can hardly help thinking that they muſt have read him, and have commented upon him. But he is ſo clear and full, though conciſe, that any commentary was certainly unneceſſary.

'The ſecond ground of belief,' p. 163, 'is *intuition*, by which I mean the mind's 'ſurvey of its own ideas, and the rela-'tions between them, and the notice it 'takes, by its own innate light, and intel-

'lective power, of what abſolutely and 'neceſſarily is, or is not, true and falſe, 'conſiſtent and inconſiſtent, poſſible and 'impoſſible, in the natures of things. It 'is to this that we owe our belief of all 'ſelf-evident truths, our ideas of the ge-'neral abſtract affections and relations of 'things, our moral ideas, and whatever 'elſe we diſcover without making uſe of 'any proceſs of reaſoning.

'It is on this power of intuition, eſſen-'tial in ſome degree or other, to all ra-'tional minds, that the whole poſſibility 'of all reaſoning is founded. To it the laſt 'appeal is ever made. Many of its per-'ceptions are capable, by attention, of 'being rendered more clear, and many 'of the truths diſcovered by it may be 'illuſtrated by an advantageous repre-'ſentation of them, or by being viewed in 'particular lights, but ſeldom will admit 'of proper proof.'

'Some truths there muſt be which can 'appear only by their own light, and

'which

'which are incapable of proof. Other-'wise nothing could be proved or known; 'in the ſame manner as if there were no 'letters, there could be no words; or if 'there were no ſimple or undefinable 'ideas, there could be no complex ideas. '—I might mention many inſtances of 'truths diſcernible no other way than '*intuitively*, which learned men have 'ſtrangely confounded and obſcured, 'by treating them as ſubjects of *reaſoning* '*and deduction*. One of the moſt impor-'tant inſtances the ſubject of this treatiſe' (viz. morals) 'affords us, and another 'we have in our notions of the neceſſity 'of a *cauſe* of whatever begins to exiſt, 'or our general ideas of *power and con-'nexion*. And ſometimes reaſon has been 'ridiculouſly employed to prove even our 'own exiſtence.'

The writers on whom I have been animadverting ſeem even to have borrowed their *language*, as well as their ideas from Dr. Price, who alſo uſes the term *common ſenſe*, but with much more propriety than they do. Of this I ſhall give two inſtances.

‘ The neceſſity of a cauſe,’ p. 31, ‘ of ‘ whatever events ariſe is an eſſential ‘ principle, a primary perception of the ‘ underſtanding; nothing being more ‘ palpably abſurd than the notion of a ‘ change which has been derived from ‘ nothing, and of which there is no reaſon ‘ to be given; of an exiſtence which has ‘ begun, but never was produced; of a ‘ body, for inſtance, that has ceaſed to ‘ move, but has not been ſtopped, or that ‘ has begun to move, without being ‘ moved. Nothing can be done to con‘ vince a perſon who profeſſes to deny ‘ this, beſides referring him to *common* ‘ *ſenſe*. If he cannot find there the per‘ ception I have mentioned, he is not ‘ farther to be argued with; for the ſub‘ ject will not admit of argument; there ‘ being nothing clearer than the point ‘ itſelf diſputed, to be brought to con‘ firm it.’

‘ Were

'Were the queſtion,' p. 62, 'what that 'perception is which we have of *number*, '*diverſity*, *cauſation*, or *proportion*; and 'whether our ideas of them ſignify *truth* 'and reality, perceived by the under-'ſtanding, or particular impreſſions, made 'by the objects to which we aſcribe them 'on our minds; were, I ſay, this the 'queſtion, would it not be ſufficient to 'appeal to *common ſenſe?*' This is not uſing the word *ſenſe* according to the technical philoſophical meaning of it, and making it, *as ſuch*, the teſt of truth; but only appealing to it as another term for a *plain underſtanding*. But it is no uncommon thing for commentators to miſtake the meaning of their author.

I thought it right to point out what ſeemed to me to be the probable ſource of what has the appearance of *truth* and *reaſon*, as alſo, perhaps, of the *miſtakes* of the writers on whom I have been animadverting; though I muſt acknowledge that I have been led to entertain a very different opinion from that of Dr. Price

Price concerning the nature and origin of the ideas above mentioned. For, inſtead of being properly *ſimple ideas*, as he conſiders them, ſeveral of them appear to me to be exceedingly *complex*, or ſubſtitutes for *deſcriptions* and *definitions*; and that at firſt view they ſeem to be ſimple for the ſame reaſon that *white* is imagined to be a ſimple colour, before we have learned how to analize it. As to the ideas of *moral right* and *wrong*, and *moral obligation*, inſtead of bearing the proper marks of ſimple and original ideas, neceſſarily reſulting from the view of any object, they appear to me exactly to reſemble ideas compounded of many parts, ſome of which are obtained earlier and others later, and which require time perfectly to coaleſce into one. The minds of children are long deſtitute of them; they are acquired very gradually; they are at firſt extremely imperfect, but grow more perfect and accurate by degrees, as their growth is more or leſs favoured by the circumſtances to which the mind is expoſed: they are ſubject to great

variations

variations in the courſe of our lives; and in ſome minds, thoſe ideas are never perfectly formed, ſome incoherent rudiments of them only being obſervable.

I am rather ſurprized that Dr. Price ſhould ſee any occaſion for ſuppoſing the faculty by which we judge of the truth of propoſitions, as diſtinct from ſimple perception, to be the ſource of ideas; ſince every perception may be reſolved into a *propoſition*, and therefore neceſſarily ſuggeſts a *truth*. If I only open my eyes, and get the idea of a *white horſe*, I as evidently perceive a *truth*, viz. that *the horſe is white*, as I perceive a truth when I have the ſentiment of *approving a generous action*; and the latter is juſt as much involved, and requires to be unfolded, before it can take the form of a propoſition, as the former. I do not therefore ſee why this very accurate reaſoner ſhould conſider *feeling* and *intuition* as two different grounds of belief, eſpecially as he aſcribes to feeling the *knowledge of our own exiſtence*, and *of the*

*ſeveral*

*ſeveral operations, paſſions, and ſenſations of our minds*, p. 162. It appears to me to be a diſtinction without a difference to make the faculty by which we judge of theſe things, to be different from that by which we judge of *all ſelf evident truths*, and get our *ideas of general abſtract affections and relations of things*, our *moral ideas*, and *whatever elſe we diſcover without making uſe of any proceſs of reaſoning;* which, however, we have ſeen that he aſcribes to *intuition*, as diſtinct from *feeling*. It equally requires an attention to what paſſes within our minds, or *reflection*, to diſcover the *operations and paſſions of our minds*, as to get ideas of *general abſtract affections and relations of things*. We may live and act under the influence of theſe ideas without knowing any thing about them; but the ſame *reflex attention* to what paſſes within ourſelves will equally diſcover them all. I do not mean to diſcuſs this ſubject with Dr. Price, it being foreign to my preſent purpoſe. Some obſervations, however, the reader will find relating to it in the *preliminary*

*preliminary Eſſay*, and more in the *Diſſertations* prefixed to my edition of *Hartley's Obſervations on man*. But for every thing of this nature I would more eſpecially refer my reader to Dr. Hartley himſelf, to whom I am indebted for almoſt all my knowledge of this ſubject.

NUM-

# NUMBER II.

## *Of* Mr. Harris's hypothesis *concerning Mind and Ideas.*

I Think it not altogether improper, in this Appendix, to take some slight notice of the hypothesis of Mr. Harris (the ingenious author of *Hermes*) relating to *mind* and *ideas*, which is so like that of Dr. Reid, that it might have been expected that he would have acknowledged some obligation to him for it; or, at least, that (as Dr. Price has done) he would have *quoted* him, as expressing sentiments so very similar to his own. The hypothesis is singular enough; but, I believe, something a-kin to that of Malebranche; though, not having studied the writings of this French philosopher, I am not able to pronounce with certainty.

If I understand Mr. Harris aright, *all our ideas are innate;* having been originally im-

impreſſed upon our minds by the Deity, and being only awakened, or called forth, by the preſence of external objects. But unleſs he could have advanced ſome more *direct evidence* for this ſyſtem than he has done, I think he is hardly to be juſtified for treating with ſo much ridicule and contempt the hypotheſis of Mr. Locke and others, that ideas are properly *produced by the actions of external objects;* there being the ſame neceſſary connection between them, as between any other cauſes and effects in nature.

'Mark the order of things,' ſays he, p. 392, 'according to their account of 'them. Firſt comes that huge body the 'ſenſible world, then this and its attri- 'butes beget *ſenſible ideas.* Then, out 'of ſenſible ideas, by a kind of lopping 'or pruning, are made *ideas intelligible,* 'whether ſpecific or general. Thus 'ſhould they admit that mind was coeval 'with body, yet till body gave it ideas, 'and awakened its dormant powers, it 'could at beſt have been nothing more 'than

'than a ſort of dead capacity; for innate
'ideas it could not poſſibly have any.'

There is a good deal of humour and fine deſcription in our author's repreſentation of the various hypotheſes of the uſe of the nerves in conveying ideas. 'At another time,' ibid. 'we hear of 'bodies ſo exceedingly fine that their 'very *exility* makes them ſuſceptible of 'ſenſation and knowledge; as if they 'ſhrunk into intellect by their exquiſite 'ſubtilty, which rendered them too deli'cate to be bodies any longer. It is to 'this notion we owe many curious inven'tions, ſuch as *ſubtle ether*, *animal ſpirits*, '*nervous ducts*, *vibrations*, &c. terms 'which modern philoſophy, upon parting 'with *occult qualities*, has found expe'dient to provide itſelf to ſupply their 'place.'

This, however, appears to me to be an evidence rather of a fine imagination in our author, than of his fairneſs, or acquaintance with the ſubject. He could not

not ſeriouſly imagine that any perſon ever ſuppoſed that *matter* was capable, by its *ſubtilty* only, of approaching to the nature of *immateriality*. All that has ever been ſuppoſed (and what facts will ſufficiently authorize) is that ideas, and their affections, are the reſult of certain impreſſions made upon the ſyſtem of the nerves and brain. To prove that this is an unphiloſophical hypotheſis, Mr. Harris muſt ſhew, not that we cannot *explain* the connection between thought and this material ſyſtem, but that there *is no ſuch connection*, and that the faculty of thinking in man can ſubſiſt without that ſyſtem; which I think he will not attempt to do.

Let us now conſider the arguments on which his own hypotheſis is founded; which, as far as I have been able to collect them out of what he has written upon the ſubject, are the following.

First, ideas are *of the eſſence of mind*, and therefore, having no relation to corporeal things, cannot be produced by them. ‘The nature of ideas,’ p. 380, ‘is not difficult to explain, if we once ‘allow a poſſibility of their exiſtence. ‘That they are exquiſitely beautiful, va‘rious, and orderly, is evident from the ‘exquiſite beauty, variety, and order, ‘ſeen in natural ſubſtances, which are but ‘their copies or pictures. That they are ‘*mental*, is plain, as they are *of the eſſence* ‘*of mind;* and conſequently no objects ‘to any of the ſenſes, nor therefore cir‘cumſcribed either by time or place.—But ‘the intellectual ſcheme,’ p. 394, ‘which ‘never forgets deity, poſtpones every ‘thing corporeal to the primary mental ‘cauſe. It is here it looks for the origin ‘of intelligible ideas, even of thoſe which ‘exiſt in human capacities. For though ‘thoſe ſenſible objects may be the de‘ſtined medium to awaken the dormant ‘energies of man’s underſtanding, yet ‘are thoſe energies themſelves no more ‘contained in ſenſe, than the exploſion ‘of a cannon in the ſpark that gave it ‘fire.’

But

But this goes upon the ſuppoſition that mind is of ſuch a nature, as that it can have no poſſible connection with matter, or be properly affected by it, which is contrary to all appearance, if the ſubject of perception and thought in man be *mind*. For, judging by the moſt obvious facts, and univerſal experience, nothing is more evident, than that the principle which we call *mind*, whether it be material or immaterial, is of ſuch a nature, that it *can* be affected by external objects, and that its perceptions correſpond to the ſtate of the corporeal ſyſtem, eſpecially that of the brain. And there is the ſame reaſon to conclude that this affection is *natural* and *neceſſary*, as that the ſound of a muſical chord is the natural and neceſſary effect of the ſtroke of a *plectrum*. If my eye be open, and a houſe be before me, I as neceſſarily perceive the idea of a houſe; or if fire be applied to any part of my body, I as neceſſarily perceive the ſenſation of burning, as ſound follows the ſtroke above mentioned. If a due attention to theſe facts obliges to alter our notions of *mind*, and *materialiſm*, the received rules of philoſophizing compel us to do it; and theſe are certainly a better authority than the mere ſpeculations of metaphyſicians, founded on no obſervations at all.

I readily admit our author's compariſon of ideas to the *exploſion of a cannon,* and of an external object to a *ſpark* that occaſions it; but I wonder that he ſhould make uſe of this compariſon, which, in effect, overthrows his whole hypotheſis. For is not the exploſion of the cannon the *mechanical effect* of the production of an elaſtic vapour, and of the increaſe of the expanſion of the air, by heat? If ideas reſult from external objects, in a manner at all analogous to the exploſion of gunpowder from the application of fire, I ſee no occaſion for having recourſe to any immaterial principle in man, or for ſuppoſing that ideas, *as ſuch,* are ſo far *of the eſſence of mind,* that they can have no relation to time or place.

Mr. Harris, moreover, admits that ſenſible objects may be a *medium to awaken the dormant energies of man's under-*

*derſtanding*, by which I ſuppoſe he means *ideas*, in the firſt inſtance, and *mental operations* afterwards. But if ſenſible objects have a natural power of *awakening* ideas, why may they not have a natural power of originally *exciting* them, in the ſame mind? Let Mr. Harris explain the difference. In both the caſes ſome *mutual action*, or *affection*, muſt be ſuppoſed.

The manner in which our author thinks that he can reduce us to the neceſſity of admitting the derivation of ideas from *mind*, rather than from *body*, is ſo curious that I ſhall tranſcribe the whole paſſage. 'Either all minds,' p. 400, 'have their 'ideas derived, or all have them original; 'or ſome have them original, and ſome 'derived. If all minds have them de-'rived, they muſt be derived from ſome-'thing which is itſelf not mind, and thus 'we fall inſenſibly into a kind of atheiſm. 'If all have them original, then are all 'minds divine, an hypotheſis far more 'plauſible than the former. But if this 'be not admitted, then muſt one mind, 'at leaſt, have original ideas, and the 'reſt have them derived. Now, ſuppoſing 'this laſt, whence are thoſe minds, whoſe 'ideas are derived, moſt like to derive 'them; from *mind*, or from *body;* from 'mind, a thing homogeneous, or from 'body, a thing heterogeneous; from 'mind, ſuch as, from the hypotheſis, has 'originally ideas, as from body, which 'we cannot diſcover to have any ideas 'at all?'

But it is no more neceſſary that bodies ſhould themſelves have ideas, in order to excite them in us, than it is neceſſary that a *plectrum* ſhould have *ſound* in itſelf, in order to excite it in a muſical chord; or that a ſpark of fire ſhould contain an exploſion, in order to produce it, by its application to gunpowder; and yet nothing but *matter* and *motion* are concerned in theſe caſes.

Secondly, Mr. Harris ſeems to think his hypotheſis neceſſary to account for the *identity of the ideas* of different minds.

'Now

'Now is it not marvellous,' p. 399, 'that 'there ſhould be ſo exact an identity of 'our ideas, if they were only generated 'from ſenſible objects, infinite in number, 'ever changing, diſtant in time, diſtant 'in place, and no one particular the 'ſame with any other?'

But is there not equal identity or diverſity in *external objects*, as there is in our *ideas* of them? It appears to me that the correſpondence is ſo ſtrict, that it amounts to a ſufficient proof of our ideas having this very origin, and no other. Men in the ſame ſituations, that is, expoſed to the ſame influences, we have reaſon to believe, will have the ſame ideas, in ſimilar ſituations, they will have ſimilar ideas, and in different ſituations they will have different ideas, and different in proportion to the difference in their ſituations.

Thirdly, our author ſuppoſes the mental origin of our ideas neceſſary to account for the correſpondence there is between the ideas of the divine mind and thofe of ours, and confequently to the communication between him and us. 'In 'fhort,' p. 395, 'all minds that are, are 'fimilar and congenial, and fo too are 'their ideas, or intelligible forms. Were 'it otherwife, there could be no inter-'courfe between man and man, or (what 'is more important) between man and 'God).—Let ideas then,' p. 399, 'be 'original; let them be connate and effen-'tial to the divine mind. If this be true, 'is it not a fortunate event, that ideas of '*corporeal* rife, and others of *mental*, '(things derived from fubjects fo totally 'diftinct) fhould fo happily coincide in 'the fame wonderful identity?'

Now, for my part, I fee no great difficulty in admitting that the divine being fhould caufe material objects to excite the very fame ideas in our minds, that might come into his fome other way. Befides, with refpect to the divine mind, I think it is fufficient, in this cafe, to plead our utter ignorance of the nature or affections

of

of it. This, however, I would obſerve, and I think it well deſerves the ſerious attention of Mr. Harris, and Dr. Reid; that if things *material* and *immaterial* be ſo very remote in their nature, the one having a relation to time and place, and the other being incapable of any relation to either, in ſo much that they cannot poſſibly affect one another (and upon this notion only can our author deny the poſſibility of external objects impreſſing our minds) and if, as he aſſerts, all minds be *ſimilar*, *homogeneous*, and *congenial*, matter can no more affect, or be affected by, the *divine mind*, than it can affect, or be affected by *ours*. Conſequently no ſuch thing can exiſt; or, if it do exiſt, it cannot have been created by God. If I be capable of drawing any conſequence, this appears to be a juſt one. Let Mr. Harris or Dr. Reid invalidate it, if they can.

As to the origin and nature of *ideas* in the divine mind, I muſt be allowed to profeſs the ſame ignorance, as of the origin or nature of his *being*.

NUM-

## NUMBER III.

*The correſpondence of the author with* Dr. Oſwald *and* Dr. Beattie, *relating to this controverſy.*

HAVING thought proper to acquaint Dr. Reid, Dr. Beattie, and Dr. Oſwald, with my intention of animadverting upon their writings, I ſent the ſame notice to each of them, at the ſame time; together with a printed copy of the preface to my third volume of the *Inſtitutes of natural and revealed religion*, and having received anſwers from Dr. Oſwald and Dr. Beattie, I have here inſerted them, with my replies, for reaſons that will ſufficiently appear in the peruſal of them.

As Dr. Oſwald ſeems to lay peculiar ſtreſs on his *ſeventh letter*, to which he refers me; and I am willing to give him all poſſible advantage, I have ſubjoined the whole of it. But if any body can think

think it to be of the leaſt uſe to his purpoſe, or that it exhibits any thing more than another ſpecimen of juſt ſuch futile declamation as I have already quoted again and again, I own he ſees more in it than I can ſee. I think it altogether unneceſſary to make any particular remarks upon it. His fifth letter alſo, I think as little ſatisfactory.

---

## *To* Dr. OSWALD.

REVEREND SIR,

THINKING it right that every perſon ſhould be apprized of any publication in which his writings are criticized, I take the liberty to ſend you a copy of a *ſheet* that will ſoon be publiſhed, in which I announce my intention to animadvert upon the principles of your *Appeal to common ſenſe*.

I am, Reverend Sir,

Your obedient humble Servant,

J. PRIESTLEY.

*London, April* 28, 1774.

REVEREND

REVEREND SIR,

I Have received your letter, announcing remarks you are to publiſh on my *Appeal to common ſenſe*, with one incloſed ſheet, containing theſe remarks for my peruſal. This, I own, is gentlemanny; but I am in no diſpoſition for accepting the challenge. I ſhall, however, point out a few things which may deſerve your notice.

Though numbers of high rank for literature in this and the preceding age have aimed at nothing beyond high probability; and though the evidence offered by Dr. Reid, Dr. Beattie, and myſelf for primary truths doth not give you ſatisfaction, you ought not to be poſitive that no other than probable evidence belongs to the ſubject; but ought to allow that higher evidence, too much neglected hitherto, and of which you have no clear conception, may poſſibly belong to the primary truths of religion.

Your

Your allusion to a lottery ticket is indecent. The utmost assurance arising from the chance of a thousand to one, is burdened with a just and rational dread of disappointment; but the evidence peculiar to the primary truths of religion leaves no room for a dread of disappointment, that can be called just or rational.

When you consult your heart, you will, I hope, find your belief of the Copernican system different from your belief of the primary truths of religion, and founded on evidence of an inferior kind. The possibility, at least, of error attends the most complete demonstration; but no such charge lies against the primary truths of religion; and this circumstance is of too great importance to be slightly passed over.

I shall not promise that the fifth letter annexed to the first volume of my Appeal on the difference between possibility, proba-

probability, and certainty, or that the laſt book of the ſame volume, on the difference between reaſoning and judging will give you ſatisfaction; but theſe are ſubjects you ought to be acquainted with, before you pronounce on the evidence which belongs to primary truths.

I ſhould be ſhy of recommending a ſecond reading of my Appeal to one who is poſitive that it contains juſt nothing; but if you will take the trouble of reading the ſeventh letter, annexed to the firſt volume, you may find that an appeal to common ſenſe in behalf of obvious truth may amount to more than people's calling one another reciprocally fools and blockheads.

I thought, and ſtill think, that divines of eminence ought to have offered ſomething more than the higheſt probability for the primary truths of religion, and that I had a right to complain of their not doing ſo, without derogating from their

their merit, or being liable to the imputation of arrogance from thoſe who are in the daily exerciſe of uttering complaints of the miſconduct of their ſuperiors.

If you know no other evidence for the primary truths of religion than the higheſt degree of probability, you cannot be juſtly blamed for offering that, and that alone, to thoſe under your care; nor have you the leaſt occaſion for quarrelling with others, who are poſſeſſed, or believe themſelves poſſeſſed, of higher evidence; and I am of opinion you may employ yourſelf with more advantage to the public by purſuing other branches of ſcience, than by deciding raſhly on a ſubject which I ſee you have not ſtudied.

When you have thought better of the matter, you will not, I preſume, chuſe to publiſh the ſheet you ſent me in the preſent form; but if you do, I ſhall expect you will do me the juſtice of publiſhing this letter along with it. I have declined

entering

entering into a controverſy, but this I inſiſt on. I am,

Reverend Sir,

Your moſt humble ſervant,

JAMES OSWALD.

*Methven, May* 12, 1774.

---

REVEREND SIR,

THE ſheet I incloſed was publiſhed exactly as it was ſent to you, about a fortnight afterwards. But if it had not, I ſhould not have thought proper to have printed your letter along with it, as I do not ſee a ſhadow of a foundation *in juſtice* for your inſiſting upon it. Dr. Reid, Dr. Beattie, and others, have juſt the ſame right, and I do not profeſs to be publiſher for all the world. The preſs is as open to you, as it is to me; and if you do not think proper to have recourſe

recourſe to it upon this occaſion, the fault is not mine. It is poſſible, however, that, in my intended publication, I may inſert this letter of yours; but if you ſaw it in the ſame light in which I do, you would requeſt that I would not.

You ſay you *ſee I have not ſtudied the ſubject;* and this letter alone proves to me that you have not thought ſufficiently upon it. But neither am I a judge of you, nor you of me. The queſtion is before the public.

Your friends, I doubt not, think very well of your writings; and on the other hand mine (among whom I have the honour to reckon a conſiderable number of the ableſt ſcholars and divines of this kingdom) think exactly as I do with reſpect to them; and think it very proper that principles which appear to them ſo falſe and dangerous ſhould receive ſome check; that, at leaſt, it may appear that *all* chriſtians are not ſo ready to abandon the only rational defence of religion. I am,

Reverend Sir, &c.

*Calne, May* 23, 1774.

I might farther obſerve with reſpect to ſome parts of Dr. Oſwald's letter, that he places our belief of the *being of God*, and of the other primary truths of religion, on the ſame foundation with that of the *external world*, the evidence of which I think I have ſhewn to be not ſtrictly ſpeaking *demonſtrative*, though it admits of no *rational doubt*. In like manner what philoſopher will ſay that the truth of the Copernican ſyſtem admits of any rational doubt, though there is a *poſſibility* that it may not be true? The being of a God I conſider as ſtrictly *demonſtrable*, which abundantly ſatisfies me with reſpect to it; though Dr. Oſwald ſays, what I have no conception of, that *the poſſibility of error attends the moſt complete demonſtration*. And when I ſuppoſe

ſuppoſe the other primary truths of religion to be as little liable to rational doubt as the truth of the Copernican ſyſtem, I think no perſon can be of opinion that I do them any injuſtice.

The reception of the primary truths of religion, and eſpecially of chriſtianity, is repreſented in the ſcriptures as depending, in ſome meaſure, upon men's previous diſpoſitions and moral characters. As our Saviour ſays, John vii. 17. *If any man will do his will, he ſhall know of the doctrine whether it be of God.* But this could not be the caſe if theſe truths were properly *ſelf-evident*, ſo that no perſon who had common ſenſe could reject them. No doubt the Scribes and Phariſees, who rejected Chriſt, had common ſenſe, as well as the twelve apoſtles; but their pride, ambition, and other vices, laid a ſtrong and undue bias upon their minds, and prejudiced them againſt him. To uſe Dr. Oſwald's own ſtyle, *I appeal to men of underſtanding*, whether it be not a more rational account of the matter, to ſay that, in all ages, men reject the primary truths of religion, natural and revealed, becauſe they are defective in *moral diſpoſitions,* rather than in *common ſenſe.*

As to the *indecency* of my alluſion to the doctrine of chances, I can only ſay that I am not ſenſible of it.

Had Dr. Oſwald's book been written in the ſame ſtrain with this letter (in which he ſays that, if I know no other evidence for the primary truths of religion than the higheſt degree of probability, I cannot be juſtly blamed for offering that and that alone) I ſhould not have quarrelled with him as he terms it, for advancing what he calls his *higher evidence.* But I appeal to the extracts that I have given, and to the whole ſtrain of his publication, if his violent and unjuſt cenſures of others, for not advancing more than they thought the nature of the caſe admitted, does not abun-

abundantly juſtify the manner in which I have vindicated their conduct, and animadverted upon his.

Dr. Oſwald is pleaſed to pay me a compliment in ſaying that '*I* might employ 'myſelf to more advantage to the public, 'by purſuing other branches of ſcience, 'than by deciding raſhly on a ſubject 'which, he ſees, I have not ſtudied.' In return to this compliment, I ſhall not affront him by telling him how very little of my time this buſineſs has hitherto taken up. If he alludes to my *experiments*, I can aſſure him than I have loſt no time at all; for having been intent upon ſuch as require the uſe of a burning lens, I believe I have not loſt one hour of ſun-ſhine on this account. And the public may perhaps be informed, ſome time or other, of what I have been doing in the *ſun*, as well as in the *ſhade*.

## Dr. OSWALD's *Seventh Letter.*

'YOU ſeem to think that a ſceptic will 'make light of the charge of folly 'that I bring againſt him; but will he 'make light of being convicted of folly 'to himſelf; for that is what I aim at? 'By appealing to common ſenſe, I do 'not truſt the cauſe of religion to a ma- 'jority of mankind, or to a certain 'number of ſelect judges, but to every 'man of ſenſe, and to the ſceptic him- 'ſelf; who, if he poſſeſſes that quality in 'any tolerable degree, will at length pro- 'nounce in favour of religion. Indeed, 'if a man is deſtitute of common ſenſe, 'or if, by diſeaſe, or otherwiſe, that cha- 'racteriſtical power of the rational mind 'is ſo impaired, as to render him inca- 'pable of diſtinguiſhing between obvious 'truth and palpable abſurdity, I do not 'ſuſtain him a judge. But that, I pre- 'ſume, is not a common caſe; for, as 'in the practice of our duty, we often 'find ourſelves urged by oppoſite affec- 'tions,

'tions, and may yield to the direction of 'either, as we chuse; so in judging on 'plain subjects, true and false sentiments 'often present themselves to our mind, 'in such a way as leaves us at liberty to 'adopt the one or the other, as we chuse. 'Have you not known persons far gone 'in folly, who still retained so much dis-'cernment, that, upon some occasions, 'they have caught themselves speaking 'nonsense, have blushed, and turned 'silent? I can recollect instances of per-'sons, in the beginning of a fever, who 'have told those about them that they 'were going to rave, and have actually 'stopped themselves; and nothing is 'more common than for those who are 'getting drunk to perceive the growing 'disorder, by the nonsense which they 'utter. If, indeed, they go on to drink, 'they will perceive it no longer, but 'turn downright fools, without the possi-'bility of being made sensible of the 'disorder.

'I always avoid charging thofe faults 'on the will, which can be fairly placed 'to the account of the underftanding; 'but cannot help thinking that fceptics 'and infidels might prevent a great deal 'of that abfurdity they run into on the 'fubject of religion: for, certain difeafed 'cafes excepted, the progrefs of folly is 'gradual, and the perfon affected may 'perceive it if he will, or may, in its 'firft approaches, be made fenfible of it, 'by the affiftance of a friend. And I 'know no greater friendfhip that can be 'done to thefe people, than to fet the 'difference between fenfe and nonfenfe 'full in their view; and am perfuaded 'that, if this good office had been done 'to mankind by the friends of religion, 'when the controverfy firft broke out, we 'had not only got rid of fcepticifm long 'ago, but alfo would have made a greater 'proficiency in ufeful knowledge than we 'have done: and I would fain hope that 'the evil may yet be redreffed, by reftor-'ing the authority of common fenfe.

'Do not you think that ſomething ought 'to be done for the honour of literature, 'and of the age in which we live? for 'what a ſhameful thing is it, that we 'ſhould be found wrangling about firſt 'principles, when diſcoveries of truths 'unknown to thoſe who came before us 'might, in all reaſon, be expected from 'a people who enjoy our advantages. 'We laugh at thoſe ſubtil diſputes of 'the ſchoolmen, which never could be 'brought to an iſſue; but are not aware 'of a conduct no leſs ridiculous, in writ-'ing volumes of controverſy about truths 'which no man of ſenſe can gainſay.

'I know your zeal for freedom of in-'quiry, and heartily agree with you; but 'cannot be reconciled to that ſilly vanity 'of maintaining either ſide of a queſtion 'by plauſible arguments; which you 'know was firſt introduced by the antient 'ſophiſts, and brought again into reputa-'tion by the Popiſh ſchoolmen, and is 'now become the chief faculty of modern 'ſceptics,

'sceptics, and not discountenanced in the 'manner it ought by men of sense and 'learning.

'How often have you and I been dis-'gusted with idle conceits, chimerical sup-'positions, and monstrous paradoxes, in 'favourite authors, which they would not 'have had the boldness to offer to the 'public, if men of learning and judgment 'had acted with the spirit which became 'them? Do you think there would be 'any harm in obliging men of genius to 'put their opinions to the trial of common 'sense before they obtruded them on the 'unthinking multitude? And if any 'should, through petulance and presump-'tion, neglect this necessary precaution, 'would it be any prejudice to the interest 'of truth, or of freedom of thought, that 'their gross adsurdities, or crude concep-'tions, were received by the public with 'that cold contempt, which they are sure 'to meet with in every circle of men of 'sense and spirit? I know no right any

'set

'ſet of men can have to inſult the com-'mon ſenſe of mankind; nor do I ſee any 'reaſon why the public ſhould bear with 'freedoms from writers of any kind, 'which one man of ſpirit would not bear 'with from another.

'After all, I am as diffident of my ſuc-'ceſs as you can be, both from a ſenſe of 'my incapacity to do juſtice to the ſub-'ject, and a ſuſpicion that mankind chuſe 'either to be entertained with ſubtil de-'bates, or to give up inquiry altogether; 'but I hope the public will take in good 'part this effort I have made,' &c.

See the remainder of this paragraph at the cloſe of my remarks on this writer.

*Aberdeen,*

*Aberdeen, May* 27, 1774.

REVEREND SIR,

I Received yours of the 28th of April inclofing a printed fheet of a *preface* not then publifhed, in which you exprefs your difapprobation of *The Effay on Truth*, and intimate your defign of animadverting further upon it. I thank you for this early notice of your intentions, and for the juftice you do me in that part of your preface where you declare that you believe me to be a fincere friend to revelation.

The Effay on Truth is fo well intended, and its principles fo well founded, that its author can have nothing to fear from the animadverfions of a man of fcience and candour. If I had not thought thofe principles true, I fhould never have given them to the world. If I did not ftill think them true, I fhould publifh my recantation to-morrow; or, if I could, to-day.

All

All that you have ſaid in your preface againſt *me* I ſhall anſwer in few words.

If your meaning, page 5th, line 19, is that '*I* repreſent common ſenſe as 'ſuperſeding almoſt all reaſoning about 'religion, natural and revealed,' you charge me with a doctrine which I do not, and never did believe, and which is no where either inſerted or implied in any thing I ever wrote.

If you mean, page 6, line 20, that *I* have ever, in word or writing, taught, or inſinuated, that '*religion in general* '(I ſuppoſe you mean natural religion) 'or chriſtianity in particular, does not 'admit of a rational and ſatisfactory 'proof,' you are, Sir, egregiouſly miſtaken in regard to my principles.—My doctrine is only this, that all reaſoning terminates in firſt principles, and that firſt principles admit not of proof, becauſe reaſoning cannot extend in infinitum; and that it is abſurd for a man to ſay, that he diſbe-lieves

lieves a firſt principle, which his conduct ſhows that he does not diſbelieve.

If you charge me with ſuppoſing, (page 7, l. 4—14) that 'the being, unity, 'attributes, and providence of God, and 'a future ſtate of retribution are either '*intuitively* certain, or certainties of the 'ſame ſort with the axioms of geometry,' you charge me with that which I never believed, or ſuppoſed, and which you will find nothing in my writings to juſtify.

You are pleaſed, Sir, to call common ſenſe *a pretended new principle.* What you may mean by the word *common ſenſe* I know not; but that which I call common ſenſe, is a *real* part of the human conſtitution, and as *old,* and as *extenſive* as human nature. I am one of thoſe, Sir, who do not like a doctrine one whit the better for its being new, nor do I think myſelf ſagacious enough to diſcover in the human mind any thing which was never diſcovered there before.

You

You honour me with the epithet *Reverend,* to which I have no title. I have told the world in my book that I am not a clergyman: but I humbly truſt I am a chriſtian; and permit me to ſay, Sir, that I have better ground to believe that my writings have hurt the cauſe of infidelity, than you can have to inſinuate the contrary, which in page 6, l. 17, in your preface you ſeem to do.

I would have anſwered you ſooner, but have been prevented by buſineſs and bad health.

I am, Reverend Sir,

Your very humble ſervant,

JAMES BEATTIE.

SIR,

SIR,

I Take the liberty to trouble you once more, to expreſs the pleaſure I have received from the great frankneſs and generoſity that are apparent in the letter you have done me the honour to write to me. I wanted no aſſurance of the goodneſs of your *intentions*, or *diſpoſition*. The ſtrain of your writings left me no room to entertain a doubt on that head. Whether the principles of your *Eſſay on truth* be *well founded*, is the only point of difference between us; and as the affair will ſoon be before the public, I ſhall not trouble you at preſent with any thing relating to it. As ſoon as my remarks ſhall be printed, and a complete copy of the book can be made up, it ſhall certainly be forwarded to you.

I alſo engage to ſhow the ſame frankneſs and openneſs to conviction that you profeſs, and a perfect readineſs to retract any thing that ſhall appear to be ill founded,

founded, or too ſevere, in my cenſure of your performance.

I may be miſtaken, and ſee things in a wrong and unfavourable light, but I am far from meaning to *cavil*, and ſhould think myſelf diſgraced by taking any ſuch advantage as unguarded expreſſions may furniſh; though ſome controverſial writers ſeem to think them juſtifiable. And, conſidering that your work is in poſſeſſion of a very high degree of the publick eſteem, that my opinions on ſome of the ſubjects of our controverſy are exceedingly unpopular, and not likely to be ever otherwiſe, and that I conſider you as a friend to the cauſe that I have myſelf moſt at heart; I hope you will have the candour to conclude, that nothing would have induced me to have entered the liſts with you on this occaſion, but a ſincere and pretty ſtrong, though perhaps a miſtaken regard to truth; the ſupport of which, how much ſoever appearances may be to the contrary, is the only method of promoting, *effectually and laſtingly*, every cauſe that is truly valuable, and worth contending for.

Confidering the very different lights in which we are apt to view the fame things, in this imperfect ftate, it were to be wifhed that we might all improve this circumftance into a leffon of mutual moderation; and, that it might teach us to think as well as we poffibly can of each other, and efpecially of the *moral influence* of our refpective opinions. To me you appear to have been exceedingly to blame in this refpect.

Perhaps no two perfons profeffing chriftianity ever thought more differently than you and I do; which may appear odd in men of liberal education, and who equally think themfelves free from prejudice, and to have been earneft and impartial in their fearch after truth. But I infer from your *writings*, and the obligation that I imagine your profefforfhip lays you under to fubfcribe the *Scotch Confeffion of faith*, that fo the cafe is. Indeed, you feem never to have had the leaft acquaintance with fuch perfons as myfelf, and my friends in this country are. But, notwithftanding this, I hope that a little reflection, aided by by the candour you ſeem to be poſſeſſed of, will ſhow you the impropriety of the ſtyle you have adopted with reſpect to ſome of the points of difference between us.

I propoſe to take the liberty, in my intended publication, to inſert the letter you have ſent me, as I am perſuaded it will do you honour; and likewiſe ſhow, that, whatever countenance your writings may *ſeem* to have given to my charge, you really diſclaim the principles I have aſcribed to you. Your teſtimony will add great weight to my obſervations on that ſubject, eſpecially in what I ſhall ſay to Dr. Oſwald.

I am truly ſorry to hear of your indiſpoſition, and wiſhing the ſpeedy and perfect re-eſtabliſhment of your health, I am, with real eſteem, SIR,

Your very humble ſervant,

J. PRIESTLEY.

*Calne, June* 29, 1774.

A CATALOGUE of BOOKS written by

# JOSEPH PRIESTLEY, LL. D. F. R. S.

AND PRINTED FOR

## J. JOHNSON, Bookfeller, at No. 72, St. Paul's Church-Yard, London.

1. THE HISTORY and PRESENT STATE of ELECTRICITY, with original Experiments, illuftrated with Copper Plates, 2d Edit. corrected and enlarged, 4to. 1l. 1s.

2. A Familiar INTRODUCTION to the STUDY of ELECTRICITY, the Second Edition, 8vo. 2s. 6d.

3. The HISTORY and PRESENT STATE of DISCOVERIES relating to VISION, LIGHT, and COLOURS, 2 vols. 4to illuftrated with a great Number of Copper Plates, 1l. 11s. 6d. in Boards.

4. A Familiar INTRODUCTION to the THEORY and PRACTICE of PERSPECTIVE, with Copper Plates, Price 5s. in Boards.

5. DIRECTIONS for impregnating Water with FIXED AIR, in order to communicate to it the peculiar Spirit and Virtues of PYRMONT WATER, and other Mineral Waters of a fimilar Nature, the fecond Edition, 1s.

6. Experiments and Obfervations on different kinds of Air, with Copper Plates, 5s. in Boards.

7. A New CHART of HISTORY, containing a View of the principal Revolutions of Empire that have taken Place in the World; with a Book defcribing it, containing an Epitome of Univerfal Hiftory, the third Edition, 10s. 6d.

8. A CHART of BIOGRAPHY, with a Book, containing an Explanation of it, and a Catalogue of all the Names inferted in it, the 4th Edition, very much improved, 10s. 6d.

9. An Effay on a Courfe of liberal Education of a Civil and Active Life; with Plans of Lectures on, 1. The Study of Hiftory and general Policy. 2. The Hiftory of England. 3. The Conftitution and Laws of England.

10. The RUDIMENTS of ENGLISH GRAMMAR, adapted to the Ufe of Schools, 1s. 6d.

11. The above GRAMMAR, with Notes and Obfervations, for the Ufe of thofe who have made fome Proficiency in the Language, the fourth Edition, 3s.

12. An

12. An ESSAY on the FIRST PRINCIPLES of GOVERNMENT and on the Nature of POLITICAL, CIVIL, and RELIGIOUS LIBERTY, the ſecond Edition, much enlarged, 5s.

13. INSTITUTES of NATURAL and REVEALED RELIGION, Vol. I. containing the Elements of Natural Religion; to which is prefixed, An Eſſay on the beſt Method of communicating religious Knowledge to the Members of Chriſtian Societies, 2s. 6d. ſewed.—Vol. II. containing the Evidences of the Jewiſh and Chriſtian Revelation, 3s. ſewed.—Vol. III. containing the Doctrines of Revelation, 2s. 6d. ſewed. —Preparing for the Preſs (May 1, 1774) the fourth and laſt Part of this Work, containing the Corruptions of Chriſtianity.

14. A Free ADDRESS to PROTESTANT DISSENTERS on the Subject of the Lord's Supper, the third Edition, with Additions, 2s.

15. The Additions to the above may be had alone, 1s.

16. An ADDRESS to PROTESTANT DISSENTERS on the Subject of giving the Lord's Supper to Children, 1s.

17. CONSIDERATIONS on DIFFERENCES of OPINION among Chriſtians; with a Letter to the Rev. Mr. VENN, in Anſwer to his Examination of the Addreſs to Proteſtant Diſſenters, 1s. 6d.

18. A CATECHISM for CHILDREN and YOUNG PERSONS, the ſecond Edition, 3d.

19. A SCRIPTURE CATECHISM, conſiſting of a Series of Queſtions, with References to the Scriptures, inſtead of Anſwers, 3d.

20. A Serious ADDRESS to MASTERS of FAMILIES, with Forms of Family Prayer, the ſecond Edition 6d.

21. A View of the PRINCIPLES and CONDUCT of the PROTESTANT DISSENTERS, with reſpect to the Civil and Eccleſiaſtical Conſtitution of England, the ſecond Edition, 1s. 6d.

22. A Free ADDRESS to PROTESTANT DISSENTERS, on the Subject of CHURCH DISCIPLINE; with a Preliminary Diſcourſe concerning the Spirit of Chriſtianity, and the Corruption of it by falſe Notions of Religion, 2s. 6d.

23. A SERMON preached before the Congregation of PROTESTANT DISSENTERS, at Mill Hill Chapel, in Leeds, May 16, 1773, on Occaſion of his reſigning his Paſtoral Office among them, 1s.

24. A Free ADDRESS to PROTESTANT DISSENTERS, as ſuch. By a Diſſenter. A new Edition, enlarged and corrected, 1s. 6d.—An Allowance is made to thoſe who buy this Pamphlet to give away.

25. Letter

25. Letters to the Author of *Remarks on ſeveral late Publications relative to the Diſſenters, in a Letter to Dr. Prieſtley*, 1s.

26. An APPEAL to the ſerious and candid Profeſſors of Chriſtianity, on the following Subjects, viz. 1. The Uſe of Reaſon in Matters of Religion. 2. The Power of Man to do the Will of God. 3. Original Sin. 4. Election and Reprobation. 5. The Divinity of Chriſt. And, 6. Atonement for Sin by the Death of Chriſt, the fourth Edition, 1d.

27. A FAMILIAR ILLUSTRATION of certain Paſſages of Scripture relating to the ſame Subject, 4d. or 3s. 6d. per Dozen.

28. The TRIUMPH of TRUTH; being an account of the Trial of Mr. Elwall, for Hereſy and Blaſphemy, at Stafford Aſſizes, before Judge Denton, &c. the ſecond Edition, 1d.

29. CONSIDERATIONS for the Uſe of YOUNG MEN, and the Parents of YOUNG MEN, 2d.

Alſo publiſhed under the Direction of Dr. PRIESTLEY.

THE THEOLOGICAL REPOSITORY;

Conſiſting of original Eſſays, Hints, Queries, &c. calculated to promote religious Knowledge, in 3 Volumes, 8vo, Price 18s. in Boards.

Among other Articles, too many to be enumerated in an Advertiſement, theſe three Volumes will be found to contain ſuch original and truly valuable Obſervations on the Doctrine of the *Atonement*, the *Pre-exiſtence of Chriſt*, and the *Inſpiration of the Scriptures*, more eſpecially reſpecting the *Harmony of the Evangeliſts*, and the Reaſoning of the Apoſtle Paul, as cannot fail to recommend them to thoſe Perſons, who wiſh to make a truly free Enquiry into theſe important Subjects.

In the Firſt Volume, which is now reprinted, ſeveral Articles are added, particularly Two Letters from Dr. THOMAS SHAW to Dr. BENSON, relating to the Paſſage of the Iſraelites through the Red Sea.

---

*E R R A T A.*

P. 103, l. 6, for *manifeſtly* read *profeſſedly*.
188, l. 5, for *acts* read *arts*.